NIYAMA

The second limb of Patañjali's Aṣṭāṅga Yoga

NIYAMA

The second limb of Patañjali's Aṣṭāṅga Yoga

YOGA COURSE PLAN

Series One - Book Three

SUSAN LODGE

PRACTICE PLANS FOR YOGA STUDENTS & TEACHERS

First published in paperback in 2020 by Sixth Element Publishing
on behalf of Susan Lodge

ISBN 978-1-912218-86-8

British Library Cataloguing in Publication Data. A catalogue record for this book is available from the British Library.

Printed in Great Britain.

Acknowledgements

I am grateful for the wisdom of the teachings of the eminent Śrī T Krishnamacharya and his son TKV Desikachar. These teachings are gradually being passed on to me by Paul Harvey who was a personal student of TKV Desikachar for over two decades. I greatly appreciate Paul's insight and clarity and his efforts to conserve the integrity of what he was taught. Thank you to my first yoga teacher and now life-long friend, Amanda Brown, for her continuing encouragement and support. Thanks also go to my students – those I see regularly and those further away.

Finally, thank you to my three grown up children, for your love, smiles and great company. You are my greatest teachers and I am thankful for the riches each of you bring to my life, this book is for you.

Contents

Preface

Close study of key yoga texts has always been part of my personal practice. I thoroughly enjoy it and have benefitted in countless ways from the profound wisdom expressed so beautifully within them. I have a particular interest in The Yoga Sūtra of Patañjali and have worked with them for more than twenty years. First, by myself, when my children were young and time and money were more limited. Then, with Paul Harvey, in small groups and personal lessons. (www.yogastudies.org). Paul has supported me towards understanding aspects of the teachings which I would never have accessed by myself and I am very grateful for his teaching.

The desire to share some of my understandings of The Yoga Sūtra of Patañjali, Upaniṣat and the Bhagavad Gītā, together with course planning skills garnered during a twenty-year career in education, spur me on to write these coursebooks. It is rewarding to support fellow yoga teachers by delivering training courses and through writing these books.

There are several more coursebooks published in this series and more to come. Each one considers a specific teaching from the Yoga Sūtra and offers adaptable plans to help develop understanding. As each teaching is grasped, we can begin to see the relationships between them and to have more appreciation of the text as a whole. I hope you find these coursebooks useful and encouraging, as you open up the wisdom of these teachings for yourself or for your students.

Ways To Work With This Course

This course is designed to be adapted according to student need. The practices included are not suitable for everyone. It is your responsibility to ensure that those chosen are appropriate and that preparation, modifications and counter postures are included. This course is not posture-focussed, here the āsana are a tool to explore and appreciate the teachings on niyama. Student understanding is secured using three complementary stages: practice, reflection and assimilation through 'off the mat' practices.

Ways of using this course to structure personal practice:

- Read the main introduction and the various translations of the sūtra.
- Record the relaxation practices on the voice recorder of your phone.
- Taking one niyama at a time – read the lesson introduction and perhaps make notes.
- Re-read translations of the sūtra, pertinent to the niyama.
- Work through the āsana, prāṇāyāma, and dhāraṇā practices, adapting for your needs. Or use the niyama information alongside your personal practice from your teacher.
- Use your voice recordings for relaxations.
- I recommend practising with each niyama until you feel you have secured some understanding.
- Repeat or progress until the course is completed.
- Support your understanding with 'off the mat' practices. For example, when studying śauca, find ways to keep the body clean with chemical free skin products, clean diet, clean sleep routines etc.

Ways of using this course to structure group teaching:

- Read the main introduction.
- Read the more detailed introductory sections on each niyama lesson.
- Make notes on the pages for personal contemplations to help clarify your understanding. Gather examples which you feel might help illuminate the teachings for your students.
- Familiarise yourself with the course overview chart so that you know where you are heading and how practices might be paced for your students.
- Select appropriate āsana and sequence them safely for your students.
- Teach the first lesson – selecting and adapting according to the needs of your group.
- Evaluate after each lesson to determine if you wish to repeat, expand or develop the teaching. I find it useful to 'hover' over each one. My students say they find repetition useful.
- You might also go 'off piste' with it. For example, when teaching śauca, introduce your students to ways of keeping the body clean with chemical free products, clean diet, good sleep routines etc.

This course has been successfully trialled as a structure for personal practice and in a range of general yoga groups. Students say they find the approach of linking teachings with practice very useful. In addition to Patañjali's Yoga Sūtra, the course references the Upaniṣat, Bhagavad Gītā, and Mahābārata, a rich foundation of texts from which the reader can confidently learn, practice and teach.

Part 1 - The Yoga Sūtra of Patañjali

Historical Context: The Yoga Sūtra of Patañjali

The Yoga Sūtra of Patañjali is a key source text on yoga and invaluable in its wisdom and practicality. Written around 300CE at a time of great philosophical investigation and debate about the nature of existence, it offers a rigorous study of human psychology. Whilst there are others, The Yoga Sūtra can be regarded as the cornerstone text of yoga. It is the one which I continually refer to in order to ensure that the practices I do, whether on or off the mat, are authentic, relevant and have substance.

Who was Patañjali?

Patañjali is a figure around whom there are many images and stories. It is useful to begin with the name. 'Pat' means to fall, and 'añjali' is the gesture of cupping the hands together - the tale of Patañjali is that he fell from heaven, into cupped hands. This special image supports the high regard in which he is held, as the writer of perhaps three important texts: The Yoga Sūtra (a study of the mind), a text on Āyurveda (the Indian science of healthcare) and a text on grammar (effective communication). Whilst there is lots we don't know about Patañjali, we do know that he was a knowledgeable, reliable and highly respected author. His works continue to inform practitioners to this day.

The Yoga Sūtra: a reliable text.

For many, many years the practices, theory and philosophy of yoga were handed down orally from teacher to student. The Yoga Sūtra of Patañjali offer us a written presentation of this yoga system and effectively link us with the reasoning and methodology of ancient practitioners.

The Yoga Sūtra was written in Sanskrit, an ancient language from Asia. The fact that it can still be read in the original Sanskrit allows scholars and students to feel confident that they are accessing it in a reasonably reliable form, the possibilities of the text having being altered or watered down over time being reduced. Various translators have, of course, brought their own biases to the work.

The sūtra style of writing was a popular form for texts such as these at the time when Patañjali was setting down the yoga system. Sūtra means 'thread' and is related to the English word 'suture'. It indicates a linking of precise teachings which together form a cohesive and integrated whole. Each individual sūtra is a short, pithy statement or aphorism. They are dense expressions with few verbs or connectives, for example in chapter one verse five when describing the movements of mind, the Sanskrit is:

vṛttayaḥ pañcatayyaḥ kliṣṭa-akliṣṭāḥ ||5||

fluctuations fivefold afflict-don't afflict

The fluctuations are fivefold and they afflict or don't afflict.

Such a concentrated and condensed style of writing, although daunting to study at times, offers many opportunities for contemplation, discussion and expansion. I visualize Patañjali's Yoga Sūtra as filigree goldwork; delicately spun and intricately constructed. Given time, space and study, they offer rich pearls of wisdom. It is possible to study this text alone, but by far the most effective method I have experienced, is to gradually unpick their meaning working closely with a knowledgeable teacher, sūtra by sūtra, and by regularly re-revisiting the text. Eventually, our understanding becomes increasingly more subtle and more comprehensive.

There are 195 sūtra in total, divided into four portions or chapters known in Sanskrit as pāda.

- Chapter one, Samādhipādaḥ (51 sūtra), describes the characteristics of a settled mind.
- Chapter two, Sadhānapādaḥ (55 sūtra), sets out the means to achieve this.
- Chapter three, Vibhūtipādaḥ (55 sūtra), first presents the remaining three internal limbs of the eight-limb system: concentration, meditation and integration. Then describes the siddhis or 'fruits' which yoga can bring.
- Chapter four, Kaivalyapādaḥ (34 sūtra), describes the state of mind known as Kaivalya, 'total freedom'. In this state the mind is completely free; from disturbances, latent impressions, habitual patterns and the guṇa. As such, it is unaffected by both external and internal influences, completely liberated.

At various points within the Yoga Sūtra, Patañjali presents ways to reduce physical and mental disturbances. For example, repetition of sacred mantra, (1:28), cultivating friendliness, compassion and dispassion (1:33), surrendering our attachment to outcomes of action (1:23) etc. But it is in chapter two that he most thoroughly details the practices which can support us, notably kriyā yoga (2:1) and aṣṭāṅga yoga (2:29). Kriyā yoga has been described as similar to 'trimming the weeds', a system of maintenance. It is not as rigorous as the eight-limb aṣṭāṅga system which is more like 'removing a thorn with a thorn'. We need to apply more acute methods to effectively remove persistent patterns which disturb us.

In 2:28 Patañjali clearly sets out the purpose of his aṣṭāṅga yoga system:

Eliminating impurity through continued practice of the eight limbs of yoga brings discernment and clear perception.
B. Bouanchaud

In 2:29 he details each of the eight āṅga (limbs/parts) which make up this method:

Yama	restraints/attitudes – how we relate towards others.
Niyama	personal observances – how we relate to ourselves.
Āsana	postures
Prāṇāyāma	extending breath
Pratyāhāra	restraining the mind's linking with the senses
Dhāraṇā	concentration
Dhyāna	meditation
Samādhi	integration/absorption

The first five limbs are classified as 'external'. They work with behaviour, attitudes, body, breath, senses and thought patterns. The aṣṭāṅga system teaches that by adopting yama and niyama we are able to develop stability in our relationships, both with others and with ourselves. We can support physical health and stability through āsana and regulate breath and energy flow through the practice of prāṇāyāma. The practice of pratyāhāra, the fifth limb, involves making efforts to reduce the minds tendency to link with the outward moving senses. The practice here is to curtail our thoughts from automatically 'going off' in the direction of information which the senses bring, e.g. dramatic images, sudden noises, tempting smells. Together the external limbs (bahirāṅga) prepare and develop our ability to direct our mind, this helps us move readily into the more focussed states of the internal limbs.

The final three limbs, dhāraṇā, dhyāna and samādhi are classified as 'antarāṅga' or internal. They work specifically with the mind/psyche. Although the antarāṅga are placed latterly by Patañjali within the eight-limbs, this is not an indication that the previous limbs of yama, niyama, āsana, prāṇāyāma and pratyāhāra must be accomplished first. Each limb is integral and ongoing in the life of those who practice yoga in its completeness. Practised together, the eight-limb system leads a student towards the goal of yoga: clarity, awareness and the freedom these bestow.

This coursebook and Patañjali

This coursebook presents a range of ways in which modern practitioners of yoga can apply the teachings from the Yoga Sūtra. It holds the teachings on settled mind from Samādhi Pādaḥ (chapter 1) as the direction, then sequences selected practices from Sādhana Pādaḥ (chapter 2) to optimise physical and energetic systems and lead towards mental clarity.

Study of yoga is most effectively done in 1-1 personal lessons with a teacher so that the work can be planned according to the individual student. However, given that a large percentage of people study yoga in group classes I present here an approach which can be effective within this group context.

Part 2 - What are Niyama?

Translations of Niyama

Niyama are the second limb of the eight-limb system described above. Commonly translated as 'personal observances' they are concerned with how we relate to ourselves and are the means we adopt to support our own peace and wellbeing.

When approaching a specific teaching within the Yoga Sūtra of Patañjali I find it useful to first consider a range of translations. By comparing and contemplating the subtle differences brought to the text by each author we can become fully immersed in the nuances of the teaching. As we practice with the translations in mind, (on niyama for example), our perception and appreciation of their relevance deepens. Our understanding becomes more discriminatory and more refined. From here, we can return to the translation which we understand to be most authoritative and 'dig deep' with that. This process of overviewing first, also enables us to become increasingly sensitive to the historical and cultural influences which have shaped particular translations.

The niyama are listed by Patañjali in sūtra 2:32, below are a range of translations:

T.K.V. Desikachar, The Heart of Yoga p 176:

Niyama comprises:

1. Cleanliness, or keeping our bodies and our surroundings clean and neat.

2. Contentment, or the ability to be comfortable with what we have and what we do not have.

3. The removal of impurities in our physical and mental systems through the maintenance of such correct habits as sleep, exercise, nutrition, work and relaxation.

4. Study and the necessity to review and evaluate our progress.

5. Reverence to a higher intelligence or the acceptance of our limitations in relation to God, the all-knowing.

Paul Harvey, www.yogastudies.org (texts and free notes page):

Self-purification, satisfaction, self-discipline, sacred study and dedication to the divine are the observances.

Alistair Shearer, The Yoga Sutras of Patañjali, P108:

The rules for living are five: Simplicity, contentment, purification, refinement, surrender to the Lord.

C. Chapple, The Yoga Sutras of Patañjali p71

Purity, contentment, austerity, self-study and dedication to Īśvara are the observances.

B. Bouanchaud, The Essence of Yoga: Reflections on the Yoga Sutra of Patañjali p114:

The five personal principles of positive action are purity, contentment; a disciplined life, study of the sacred texts, and worship of God.

Sri Swami Satchidananda, The Yoga Sutra of Patanjali p119:

Niyama consists of purity, contentment, accepting not causing pain, study of spiritual books and worship of God (self-surrender).

Why Practice Niyama?

Srivatsa Ramaswami and A.G. Mohan describe yama as the 'don'ts' and niyama as the 'dos', without which 'there can be no meaningful yoga practice possible', Srivatsa Ramaswami, Yoga Beneath the Surface, p3.

The adoption of yama and niyama are prerequisites for the practice of yoga and are required to be developed continually. 'Constant remembrance' is encouraged through daily review. Patañjali taught that if we do not practice yama and niyama our efforts with the other limbs, (āsana for example), will not be fruitful and we will continue in the cycle of ignorance and pain:

'an angry young man, without deliberate attention and effort, will end up an angry old man, despite all other efforts'.

S. Ramaswami, Yoga Beneath the Surface p.5

The Benefits of Niyama

The outcomes of niyama are presented in YS 2:40-45. The chart below groups several translations of each.

2:40 Śauca - external cleanliness - body and environment

When cleanliness is developed it reveals what needs to be constantly maintained and what is eternally clean. What decays is the external. What does not is deep within us. Our overconcern with and attachment to outward things, which is both transient and superficial is reduced. TKV Desikachar

From cleanliness, disdain for own body, non-association with others.
Paul Harvey

Purity protects one's body and brings nonphysical relationships with others.
B. Bouanchaud

Simplicity destroys identification with the body, and brings freedom from contact with other bodies. Alistair Shearer

From purity arises dislike for one's own body and noncontact with others.
C. Chapple

2:41 Śauca - internal cleanliness - mind

In addition, one becomes able to reflect on the very deep nature of our individual selves, including the source of perception, without being distracted by the senses and with freedom from misapprehension accumulated from the past.
TKV Desikachar

From purity of clarity, open-mindedness, one-pointedness, mastery of the senses and capability for seeing the essence.
Paul Harvey

Then purity, clarity, and well-being of the spirit come to flower, as well as concentration, mastery of the eleven sense organs, and perception of the inner being.
B. Bouanchaud

Purity of mind, cheerfulness, mastery of the senses, one pointedness and readiness for self-realization follow. Alistair Shearer

And purity of sattva, cheerfulness, one-pointedness, mastery of the senses, and fitness for the vision of the self. C. Chapple

2:42 Saṃtoṣa - contentment

The result of contentment is total happiness. TKV Desikachar

From contentment, unsurpassed happiness is attained. Paul Harvey

Contentment brings supreme happiness. B. Bouanchaud

From contentment unsurpassed happiness is gained. Alistair Shearer

From contentment unsurpassed happiness is obtained. C. Chapple

2:43 Tapas - self-purification

The removal of impurities allows the body to function more efficiently. TKV Desikachar

From self-discipline, impurities diminish and accomplishment in the body and senses. Paul Harvey

By eliminating impurity, a disciplined life brings perfection and mastery to the body and the eleven sense organs. B. Bouanchaud

By purification, the body and the senses are perfected. Alistair Shearer

From austerity arises the destruction of impurity and the perfection of the body and senses. C. Chapple

2:44 Svādhyāya - self-study

Study, when it is developed to the highest degree, brings one close to higher forces that promote understanding of the most complex. TKV Desikachar

From self-study, total joining together with chosen deity. Paul Harvey

Union with the chosen divinity comes from the study of self through the sacred texts. B. Bouanchaud

Refinement brings communion with the desired celestial being. Alistair Shearer

From self-study (arises) union with the desired deity. C. Chapple

2:45 Īśvara Praṇidhānā - surrender

Reverence to God promotes the ability to completely understand any object of choice. TKV Desikachar

From dedication to the lord, accomplishment in integration. Paul Harvey

Contemplation and its powers are attained through worship of God. B. Bouanchaud

From surrender to the Lord, the state of samadhi is perfected. Alistair Shearer

Perfection in samadhi (arises) from dedication to Īśvara. C. Chapple

The translations cited above explain how niyama can support a practitioner's development. At the simplest level these practices give us a more distanced perspective so that we can become less entangled in 'stuff'. Gary Kraftsow relates that TKV Desikachar used to say: 'Our fundamental dharma is to be happy', explaining that the main purpose of yoga is to 'surface our saṃskāra'. Sustained yoga practice reveals behaviours and ways of thinking which would be better reduced or removed. Once we recognise them, we can take action.'

Each time I revisit these teachings on saṃskāra, I am reminded of a period when I was teaching full time in school and had three young children. Life was so hectic that for a couple of years running I hadn't had time to buy a favourite colleague a birthday card. I was too busy to be kind and it didn't feel good. In the same year I'd begun practising yoga. Within the space of my practice I was waking up to the fact that all the 'doing' wasn't satisfying. Things needed to change. Through better self-care, more order, valuing what we already had, reflecting on yoga teachings and understanding more of the 'bigger picture', things gradually improved. We made adjustments and life began to have more balance, perspective and peace.

This example demonstrates how the practice of niyama can support us. Through simplification and purification, we create the conditions where we have more space, understanding and contentment. Within this space there is the opportunity for us to link to our 'essence', to be in touch with pure awareness and joy, 'sat-cit-ānanda. When we are so completely caught up in the world that we can't see how things really are, connection with our true nature is not possible. The chart below illustrates how the beneficial outcomes of niyama help us towards greater awareness. Each niyama will be explored in turn within the study units which make up this course.

Part 3 - Niyama Course Overview

Sūtra In Sanskrit	Meaning	Beneficial outcomes
Śauca – purity (external) Sūtra: 2:40 śaucāt-sva-aṅga-jugupsā paraiḥ asaṃsargaḥ	**Śauca** – purity of body and personal environment From cleanliness, disdain for own body, non-association with others.	Through systematic care of the body and personal environment we reduce the influence of the guṇa - rajas and tamas. The system is more sattva, so there is greater balance and stability. We become more aware of what is impermanent, in ourselves and others. Through śauca we become less pre-occupied and attached to the physical and more accepting of the process of aging and death. Then, space opens up for us to consider the finer aspects of our existence.
Śauca - purity (internal) Sūtra 2:41 sattva-śuddhi-saumanasya-eka-agrya-indriya-jaya-ātma-darśana-yogyatvāni ca	**Śauca** - purity of mind From purity of clarity, open-mindedness, one-pointedness, mastery of the senses and capability for seeing the essence.	Through śauca the mind also becomes more purified, peaceful, balanced – more sattvic. It maintains focus, becomes less distracted by information coming in through the senses and has greater clarity. Consequently, we have more open attitudes and greater awareness of prejudices. We are motivated to give the mind good 'food-for-thought' and more able to direct it where we want it to go. The capability of recognising our true, unchanging nature is an outcome.
Saṃtoṣa - contentment Sūtra 2:42 saṃtoṣāt-anuttamaḥ sukha-lābhaḥ	**Saṃtoṣa** - contentment From contentment, unsurpassed happiness is attained.	The quality of happiness we experience when we are content is superior to a happy mood. It is deeper, more sustained, and arises as a result of a connection we make with our essence.

Tapas – self-purification Sūtra 2:43 kāya-indriya-siddhiḥ aśuddhi-kṣayāt-tapasaḥ	**Tapas** – self-purification From self-discipline, impurities diminish and accomplishment in the body and senses.	Informed discipline allows us to reduce impurities in many forms: sugar, bad habits, gossip, sleep, etc. Tapas is also being comfortable within the discomfort of discipline and staying with our efforts to adopt the eight limbs of yoga. Through careful discipline we are able to establish a healthful body and mind and create the conditions for fruitful contemplation.
Svādhyāya – self-reflection Sūtra 2:44 svādhyāyāt-iṣṭa-devatā-saṃprayogaḥ	**Svādhyāya** – self-reflection From self-study, total joining together with chosen deity.	A prime function of yoga practice is to allow the surfacing of saṃskāra (habits/latent impressions) so that we can address them. Self-study assists us in this. Through self-reflection with reference to the teachings of special texts, we are able to link with higher understandings which support us.
Īśvara Praṇidhānā - surrender to the divine. Sūtra 45: samādhi-siddhiḥ īśvara-praṇidhānāt	**Īśvara Praṇidhānā** – surrender. From dedication to the lord, accomplishment in integration.	When we recognise the truth of our place within the wider system and acknowledge the things which can be influenced and the things which can't, we can reach a state of greater harmony and union both internally and externally. When we regularly contemplate divine qualities, we can become integrated with those qualities.

Take time to reflect…

Jot down any personal thoughts, questions, experiences and ideas to help clarify your understanding of the teachings of niyama…

Lesson Focus	Orientation: breathing observations.	Āsana	Prāṇāyāma	Dhāraṇā	Relaxation
Study 1 Śauca: purity/ cleanliness External purity: of body and personal environment.	Semi supine pose: 1.Observe soft tissue movement in abdomen using hands. 2.Observe bony tissue movement in pelvic bowl.	Āsana as support for physical cleansing by assisting systemic health and stability.	Explore supports for sitting. 1.Observe directional flow of breath. 2.Lengthen exhales within range.	Focus: purity of body.	Guided visualisation: waterfall. Relaxation taking awareness down through the body with 'cleansing waves' of water.
Study 2 Śauca: purity/ cleanliness Internal Purity: of mind.	Balāsana - Child's Pose: 1.Observe soft tissue movements, sternum to pubis. Then back of pelvis, buttocks and hips. 2.Observe bony tissue movement in the pelvis.	Āsana as support for mental cleansing by directing attention, quietening mind movements.	1.Standing: Ujjāyī breath. 2.Seated: observe directional flow of breath. 3.Develop Ujjāyī.	Focus: mental purity	Guided visualisation: cleansing white light. Relaxation using light to release impurities in the body and release negative thought patterns.
Study 3 Saṃtoṣa: contentment.	Balāsana – Child's Pose: Observe how the breath moves the pelvic floor.	Use of static postures to explore stability, ease and satisfaction.	1.Seated: Revise ujjāyī breathing. 2. Use ujjāyī, observe directional flow of breath. 3. Lengthen exhale within range.	Focus: quotes on contentment.	Relaxation - releasing muscular tension and developing contentment, gratitude and optimism.

Study 4 Tapas: self-purification, heat, discipline.	Semi supine pose: Observe breath movement in the pelvis, lumbar, thoracic and cervical vertebrae.	Āsana as medium for awareness of sustaining appropriate discipline.	1.Seated: Revise ujjāyī breathing. 2. Use ujjāyī, observe directional flow of breath. 3. Lengthen exhale within range.	Focus: Sthira and sthiti. Remaining within consistent healthful habits.	Guided visualisation: healthy meal. Relaxation using heat / warmth and nutrition. Visualise nourishment of the body through healthy food.
Study 5. Svādhyāya: self – study.	Semi supine pose: Observe breath movements in the hips and femurs.	Develop self-awareness in āsana by observing attitudes to practice.	1.Teach breath counting technique. 2. Ujjāyī + breath counting technique. 3. Use ujjāyī, breath counting + lengthening exhale.	Focus: self-understanding	Relaxation using teachings from special texts. Hold a short, gentle, teaching in given parts of the body.
Study 6 Īśvara-praṇidhānā: surrender to the divine.	Semi supine pose: Observe breath movements in the chest: at the sternum, front ribs, side ribs and clavicles.	Explore the attitude of surrender in selected āsana	1.Revise breath counting technique. 2. Breath counting and ujjāyī. 3. Teach Anuloma Ujjāyī	Focus: qualities of Īśvara.	Relaxation using surrender. Recap each niyama. Acknowledge and respect personal efforts to secure them, then surrender effort.

Take time to reflect…

Jot down any personal thoughts, questions, experiences and ideas…

Are there any other practices which you would include?

Where would you place them?

Part 4: Practice Plans

Study 1 - Understanding Śauca

Sūtra 2:40 śaucāt-sva-aṅga-jugupsā paraiḥ asaṃsargaḥ ||40||

From cleanliness, disdain for own body, non-association with others.
Paul Harvey

Study 1 - Understanding Śauca (External) 75 min practice

Introduction 5 mins

Patañjali's eight limb yoga system is comprised of: yama, niyama, āsana, prāṇāyāma, pratyāhāra, dhāraṇā, dhyāna and samādhi. Niyama are the second limb of a system designed to bring about the containment of fluctuations in the psyche and allow us to come into the state of yoga.

The Sanskrit 'niyama' has been translated most frequently as 'observances' and more recently by Ranju Roy and David Charlton as 'self-care', (Embodying the Yoga Sutra 2019). Niyama are guides for how we might positively relate towards ourselves. The five niyama are śauca, saṃtoṣa, tapaḥ, svādhyāya and īśvara-praṇidhānā. This first lesson contemplates śauca – cleanliness or purity. We consider why we are advised to practise cleanliness and how the practise of cleanliness can support us.

Sūtra 2:32: śauca-saṃtoṣa-tapaḥ svādhyāya-īśvara-praṇidhānāni niyamāḥ

Cleanliness, contentment, self-discipline, self-study and dedication to the lord are the observances. Paul Harvey

The Sanskrit root of śauca is 'to shine' or 'gleam'. Śauca is usually explained in relation to the body, for example, it is often referenced when yoga practitioners are encouraged to keep the body healthy through a 'clean' diet and good hygiene. This way of interpreting śauca is useful to begin with and is certainly part of the practice, however, śauca is much more than this.

The practice of śauca is fundamentally about supporting the conditions for sattva guṇa to arise. Sattva guṇa is one of three constantly fluctuating energetic constituents (guṇa) of nature, in this case a constituent of our body and mind. The three constituents are: rajas (quickness, changeability), tamas (heaviness, stability, dullness) and sattva (lightness and equilibrium). When sattva guṇa predominates it brings a sense of spaciousness and balance which helps us feel steady and clear. By taking regular care of our personal environment, body and mind, by making efforts with purification, we can encourage the conditions for sattva guṇa to be present. The steadiness and clarity which result bring us closer to the state of yoga.

Patañjali separates the outcomes of śauca into two distinct aspects. The external aspect, which is concerned with a person's environment and body and the internal aspect which is concerned with the mind. This first lesson will look at the external aspects.

External Śauca - Environment

An everyday example of the practice of śauca with respect to our environment might be when we tidy our bedroom or shed. If we tidy at a surface level, the space feels a little calmer, more pleasant. But if we deep clean the room, even 'Marie Kondo' it, we create more significant change. Feelings of things 'crowding in' and the resultant confusion are replaced by a sense of openness, pleasantness and comfort. We move from chaos to order and it feels good. Also, by reducing the things we don't need we are more aware of what we do need. Cleanliness and order bring satisfaction and clarity. In this uncluttered environment everything is in place to help us smoothly accomplish the things we consider worthwhile.

'In space cometh grace.' John Heywood

External Śauca - Body

The process of taking care of ourselves physically evolves in a similar way. We nurture our general health through good diet, good sleep and exercise - equivalent to the 'general tidy up' described above. When we supplement this with sustained practice of āsana, prāṇāyāma, dhāraṇā and perhaps chanting, the outcomes are more profound. The practices create energetic change, we are cultivating sattva within our system. Lightness, ease and spaciousness become our experience within the body.

In 2:40 Patañjali describes the first outcome of 'external śauca':

śaucāt-sva-aṅga-jugupsā paraiḥ asaṃsargaḥ ||40||

From cleanliness, disdain for own body, non-association with others.
Paul Harvey

'Disdain for one's own body' can appear harsh and unrelatable to a twenty first century, Western reader. It is difficult to grasp, given the 'lightness, ease and spaciousness' of sattva guṇa which we can experience from practising. Swami Satchidananada's translation as 'disgust' even more so:

2:40 *By purification arises disgust for one's own body and for contact with other bodies.*
Swami Satchidananda

This sūtra is a good example of how studying the Yoga Sūtra with a teacher really helps. During a personal lesson with Paul Harvey he explained that although the language of 'disgust' or 'disdain' appears extreme, this degree of separation from over-concern with the body is required, due to the strength of our attachment to it. Evidence of this is clear – media advertisements exploit our concerns around the age, appearance, condition, decline and longevity of our physical bodies. The Yoga Sūtra encourage us towards a more detached relationship with it. TKV Desikachar's translation is helpful:

2:40 *When cleanliness is developed it reveals what needs to be constantly maintained and what is eternally clean. What decays is the external. What does not is deep within us.* TKV Desikachar

Through the clarity which arises from the practices of yoga, we become aware of what decays and what doesn't. Whilst taking good care of the body, we observe and accept the natural order of aging. It greatly assists our efforts to remain steady if we can accept these changes. By accepting the aging-process we become less pre-occupied with our body and those of others. A.G. Mohan explains śauca like this:

Mastery over the external cleanliness of the body, makes the yogi realize that it is unclean by nature.

As a result, he develops a feeling of disgust towards his body. Therefore, the desire to touch others, ceases.

Some translators are even more specific in their interpretation and householder practitioners may find these difficult to engage with:

2:40 *As a result of purity there arises indifference toward the body and disgust for physical intercourse with others.*

Swami Prabhavananda and Christopher Isherwood

Perhaps the translation by David Charlton and Ranju Roy in Embodying the Yoga Sutra (p 227) is more relatable for twenty first century, Western yoga students:

2:40 *From self-care arises a lack of obsession with our own bodies and a reduction of infatuation with those of others.*
David Charlton and Ranju Roy

In short, alongside recognising the transient condition of our own bodies, we come to an understanding of the temporary attractions of others.

The purpose of this first practice is to direct your attention away from the everyday things going on in your life and onto your body and breath. We encourage the mind to become one-pointed by directing it towards how the breath moves the pelvis. These movements are very subtle and require close attention.

To clarify your understanding of how your breath is currently working, after the practice you may wish to make notes on the movements you observe. You might also like to identify areas of your body where movement feels restricted. The page opposite is offered for you to record what you discover.

Lay down in semi -supine, toes pointing forwards, knees above ankles.

Anchor the back of the pelvis into the floor. Ease the spine long, by stretching away through the crown of the head.

As much as is possible for you today, allow the breathing to be soft, relaxed, unrestricted and spontaneous.

Breathe through the nostrils, but if this is uncomfortable, through the mouth and nostrils.

Observing Soft Tissue Movement. 4-6 breaths

Place the hands on the abdomen, long middle fingers at the level of your navel, palms spread.

Observe through your hands, the movements in the abdomen created by the breath.

Notice how your abdomen moves as you breathe in and out.

Watch the movement of the soft tissue in the abdomen.

Notice how much movement there is.

Notice the direction of movement.

Notice the strength of movement.

Observing Bony Tissue Movement. 6-8 breaths

Now let your arms relax down alongside your body, a little distance away from your hips, palms turned up.

Take your attention to the bony structure of your pelvis. The triangular sacrum at the centre of the back of the pelvis, the iliac bones either side and the large lumbar vertebrae rising out from the pelvis.

Hold your attention in this area and observe any subtle movements in the bony pelvic bowl as you breathe.

Perhaps you notice a slight tilting forward in the pelvis as you inhale, lumbar vertebrae lifting away from the floor.

Perhaps you notice a slight releasing back as you exhale.

This subtle and spontaneous movement into a gentle backbend as you inhale and release as you exhale is the basis of the relationship between breath with āsana in this course. We open into backbends on inhalations and release into forwards bends on exhalations.

Let the observing of the pelvis gradually release.
Let your attention rest at your sternum.

Notes on Breath Observations

Where did you feel breath movements?

What were the directions?

What were the qualities of your breathing?

Rough/smooth? Long/short? Fast/slow? Consistent/changing? Effortful/effortless?

Śauca: cleanliness - external

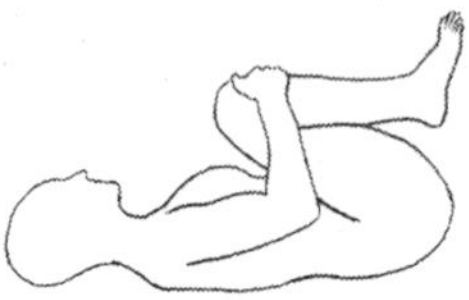

1. Apānāsana - dynamic

Exhale draw knee to chest. Inhale release.

x4 R + L. x4 both legs

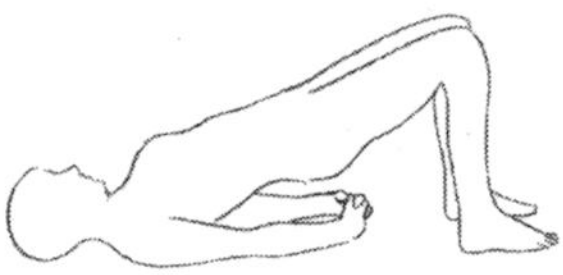

2. Dvipāda Pīṭham - dynamic

Inhale lift pelvis, exhale lower. Arms still. x4

Inhale lift pelvis and arms, exhale lower x4

Static: stay lifted 2-4 breaths

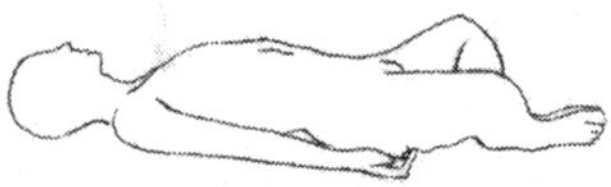

3. Supta baddha koṇāsana - static

Bend knees over chest, part them. Circle x4 both ways.

Static: Lower feet, open knees to floor, stay 4 breaths

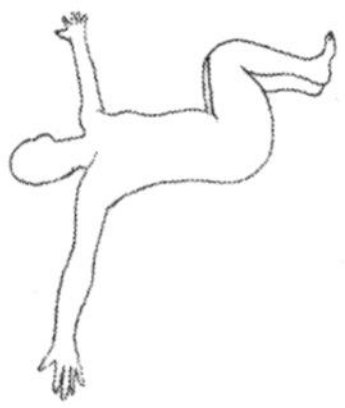

4. Jaṭhara parivṛtti - dynamic

Exhale lower legs half way to floor x2 R + L

Exhale lower legs to floor x2 R + L

Counterpose with Apānāsana

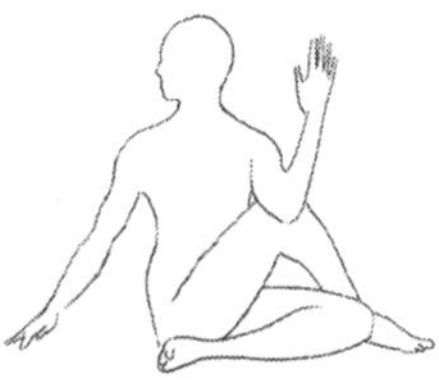

5. Ardha Matseyendrāsana - dynamic

Gradually rotate to R 4 breaths. L 4 breaths

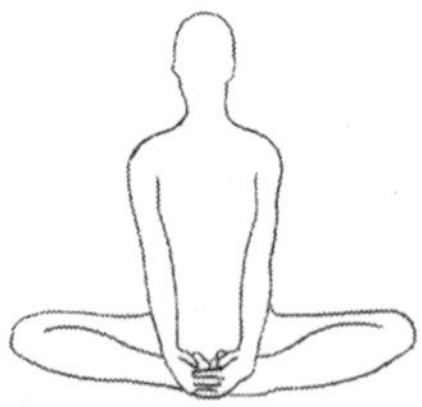

6. Baddha Koṇāsana - static

Release knees open to supports.
Stay 4 breaths.

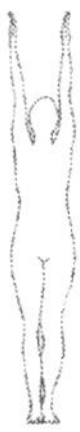

7. Tāḍāsana - dynamic

Start samasthiti – stay 4 breaths

Then inhale raise arms, exhale lower x4

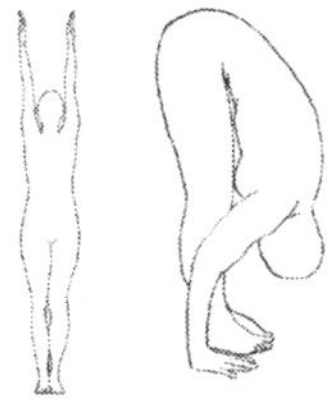

8. Ardha Uttānāsana /Uttānāsana - dynamic

Inhale raise arms, exhale fold forward
to 90°/support x4

Inhale raise arms, exhale fold forward
to fullest personal point x4

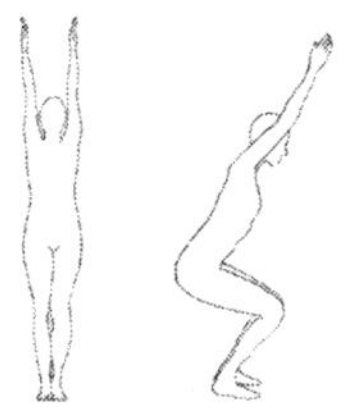

9. Ardha Utkaṭāsana/Utkaṭāsana - dynamic

Inhale raise arms exhale squat half way x4

Inhale raise arms exhale squat full way x4

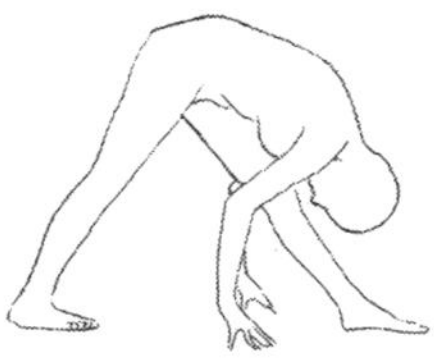

10. Parśva Uttānāsana - dynamic

Inhale raise arms above head

Exhale fold forward over front leg x4 R + L

Counterpose with Uttanāsana

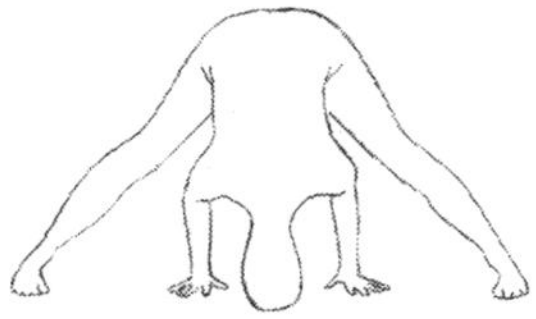

11. Prasārita Pāda Uttānāsana – static

Inhale raise arms, exhale fold forwards to support or floor.

Stay 4-6 breaths.

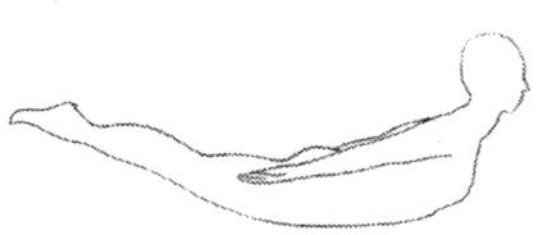

12. Śalabhāsana – dynamic.

Inhale lift arms and legs, Exhale lower x4

Counterpose with Balāsana. Come to seated.

Take a seated position with support if required. Use a chair, kneeling stool, or blocks to establish an uplifted spine and a way for the hips to be positioned above the knees for stability.

1.Place both palms flat on the upper chest. Observe the inhale as it moves first into the chest, then descends into the lower lobes of the lungs.
6 breaths

2. Place both palms on the abdomen. Observe the exhale releasing.
6 breaths

Gently draw the abdominal muscles in to support the exhale up and out at the nostrils.

3. R palm on chest, L palm on abdomen, watch the breath - in at chest, out from abdomen. 6 breaths

4. Lengthen the exhalation without strain. 4 breaths.

5. Release longer exhalations. Observe the natural length. In at chest out from abdomen. 4 breaths

The focus for this practice is cleanliness/purity of the body and personal environment.

Choose an object which signifies purity of body and environment, will engage your attention and feel positive. For example, a sparkling glass of clean water, an image of a mountain stream, a piece of fruit, a white cloth or cup. Have it ready for your concentration practice.

Come into a comfortable seated position on a chair, blocks or kneeling stool.

Rest the lengthened arms onto the legs, hands in Jñāna mudrā.

Lower the eyes and observe your breath settling into a gentle, regular rhythm. 4 breaths

Be aware of the cleansing function of the exhalation removing impurities from the circulatory system. 4 breaths

Now let your eyes rest on your chosen 'pure' object.

Let your full concentration remain on this object as you sit.

If your attention wanders, simply bring it back to the object and focus again. 3/4 mins

Begin to let your attention gradually move away from the object and back to your breathing.

Gently bring your hands into your lap, R palm resting on top of L. Let your eyes slowly re-focus.

Come out of the practice.

External Śauca - Waterfall Visualisation

Come into a comfortable semi-supine position. Feel the back of the pelvis settling into the mat.

Anchoring the pelvis, feel the spine is as long and free as it can be. Release it and allow it to settle into the mat.

Let the palms turn gently upwards to face the ceiling. Let the upper arms rotate softly upwards and outwards so that the shoulders relax back and the chest gently opens. Hands are soft, fingers lightly curled.

Let the legs stay in supine if you enjoy this support into your back, or slowly stretch them out.

Allow the heels to gently release into the mat, toes softly turning outwards.

Feel that the centre point at the back of the head is resting perfectly, the head fully supported by the floor.

Enjoy the whole body releasing down. Gently adjust any points of discomfort.

Now begin to visualise that you are lying on a grassy area by a cool pool. There is a small waterfall and you can hear the sounds of water flowing over rocks and splashing into the pool beneath.

It is a hot, sunny day and the suns' rays are softly warming your skin.

The grass is soft and lush beneath you and the ground is dry.

A light breeze is drifting over you and you can hear the soft sounds of the breeze moving through bushes and trees. You feel soft and warm and peaceful.

After a while you begin to feel a little hot and decide to go into the pool.

You walk to the water's edge and climb easily down the rocky stepping-stones.

You sink gently into the water to the depth you enjoy. The water is cool and refreshing as you wade towards the edge of the pouring waterfall.

You ease your left side under it and let the water cascade in a cool shower over your left shoulder, your left upper back, your left chest. The water eases down over your whole left side cleansing, refreshing, invigorating.

Now you slowly turn, allowing your right side to edge into the flow.
The coolness of the water slides over your right shoulder, your right upper back, your right chest. The water cleanses, cools and energises your whole right side.

If you enjoy it, let your whole body come under the flow of water, let it stream over your head and drench your body. Feel cleansed, refreshed, alive. Soothed and cool, you feel ready to leave the pool.

You wade softly back to the bank and climb easily up the rocks to the grassy bank.

You lay out on the grass or rest against a tree trunk in the shade. Enjoy the warm Summer air gradually drying your skin. You relax quietly, feeling cleansed, refreshed and purified. Your whole body feels fresh and at ease and all is well in your world.

Now begin to let this image fade.

Let the feelings of relaxation and ease stay with you as you begin to become more aware of yourself lying here resting.

Let your breath deepen. Make small movements in the hands and feet.

Let the movements grow and gradually reawaken in the ways that you enjoy.

Rest onto your side for a few breaths before coming up to sitting.

Off the Mat Practices

Keep your personal spaces clean and tidy.

Thoroughly clean out one drawer or cupboard. Continue round your home if you feel motivated to do so.

Drink two litres of pure water each day.

Avoid excessive use of stimulants such as tea, coffee, sugar, spicy foods.

Avoid excessive use of intoxicants such as cigarettes, alcohol, drugs.

Reduce, then remove, processed foods from your diet.

Use chemical free skin products including aluminium free deodorants.

Establish regular sleep habits.

Create self-care rituals, for example, bathe and oil your body before personal āsana practice.

Contemplations…

I am committed to consistently taking care of my body.

I support my body to be cleansed and pure.

I release poor eating habits such as…

My food is fresh and in its natural form.

I live in harmony with nature.

Gītā 17.14 *'Purity, honesty, continence and non-violence: these are the disciplines of the body.'*

'Muddy waters let stand, becomes clear.' Lao Tzu

Take time to reflect...

Which practices felt 'cleansing'?

In what ways did they feel beneficial?

How are your habits changing in relation to cleanliness of body?

How are your habits changing in relation to cleanliness of your personal environment?

What sources of support would help you sustain this and perhaps develop it further?

Study 2 - Understanding Śauca

Sūtra 2:41 sattva-śuddhi-saumanasya-eka-agrya-indriya-jaya-ātma-darśana-yogyatvāni ca ||41||

From purity of clarity, open-mindedness, one-pointedness, mastery of the senses and capability for seeing the essence.
Paul Harvey

Study 2 - Understanding Śauca (Internal) 75 mins practice

Introduction 5 mins

The importance of śauca within the five niyama is notable as Patañjali describes two distinct sets of outcomes in separate sūtra, the remaining niyama have only one sūtra each. In lesson one we considered the external aspect of śauca relating to a person's environment and body. Here we explore the practice of śauca as it relates to the mind.

Most students come to yoga through a physical practice, perhaps joining an āsana class or having personal lessons to sustain good health, recover from injury or address illness. The physical work leads to enhanced strength and flexibility, ease of movement and increased confidence. We feel better. This encourages us towards a more regular practice which brings change at an energetic level. More frequent states of sattva guṇa characterised by lightness, spaciousness and ease, arise in the system. Sustained practice, perhaps including a wider range of techniques such as prāṇāyāma, dhāraṇā and chanting, further supports sattva and over time we observe more subtle changes - in the qualities of mind. Patañjali lists these improvements in 2:41 as greater optimism, concentration, less susceptibility to attractions coming in through the senses and refinement of our ability to perceive our Essence.

2:41 *From purity of clarity, open-mindedness, one-pointedness, mastery of the senses and capability for seeing the essence.* Paul Harvey, yogastudies.org

In other words, purity or cleanliness of mind brings about mental clarity. With practice, we begin to recognise aspects of life which are subject to change such as our moods, our beliefs, opinions, fashions and trends. We come to understand that everything is changing and that due to their impermanence, they are not as significant as we once thought. Far from being depressing, this 'waking up' can feel light and optimistic. Gradually, the things we were preoccupied with fall away and there is a release from the endless spiralling of expectations and goals. The 'bigger picture' emerges and then, if we wish, we are free to take as priorities: a contemplation of our ongoing, essential nature, consideration of our place in the world and how we can live well within it. As Dave Charlton and Ranju Roy translate, the practice of internal (mental) śauca fosters the development of:

a clear mind, positive attitude, focus, control of the senses and a fitness for a deeper experience of the Self. Embodying the Yoga Sūtra p231

The purpose of this practice is to orientate your attention and to observe your body and breath.

We began lesson one using a semi-supine position to observe how the breath moves the soft tissue in the abdomen and the pelvis. In this lesson we will use Balāsana – Child's Pose to observe.

After practice you might like to record the qualities of your movements on the page opposite.

As much as is possible today allow your breathing to be soft, relaxed, unrestricted and spontaneous. Preferably through the nostrils, but if this is uncomfortable, through the mouth and nostrils.

Come to high kneeling, then slowly ease your pelvis back and down towards your feet. Use any props you need for support. Let the lower spine stretch back as you lower, then settle. Let the head be supported.

Let the arms lay alongside the legs, or stay forwards, whichever is most comfortable.

Bring your attention to the area between the base of the sternum and the pubic bone.

Notice how the soft tissue of your abdomen moves in Balāsana as you breathe in and out. 4 breaths

Notice how much movement there is.

Notice the direction of movement. Notice the qualities of movement.

Now watch the movement of soft tissue in the back of the pelvis, buttocks and hips. 4 breaths

Notice how much movement there is.

Notice the direction of movement. Notice the qualities of the movement.

Now watch the movement of the bony pelvic girdle. 4 breaths

Notice how much movement there is.

Notice the direction of movement. Notice the qualities of the movement.

Gradually allow these observations to release and let your attention come to your forehead resting.

Bring your hands alongside your shoulders and use your arms to push your back gently up.

Notes on Breath Observations

How were the breath movements between the sternum and pubis?

How were the breath movements in the soft tissue of the back of pelvis, buttocks and hips?

How were the breath movements of the bony pelvis in Balāsana?

What were the qualities of your breathing in this position?
Rough/ smooth? Long/short? Fast/slow? Consistent/changing? Effortful/effortless?

How does your breathing in Balāsana differ to that in semi-supine?

Select from the āsana below, adding appropriate modifications and counter postures according to student need and ability.

Śauca: cleanliness - internal

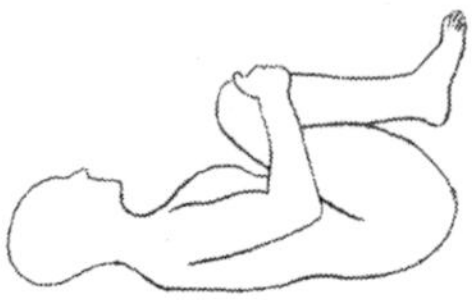

1. Apānāsana - dynamic

Exhale draw knee to chest. Inhale release.

x4 R + L. x4 both legs

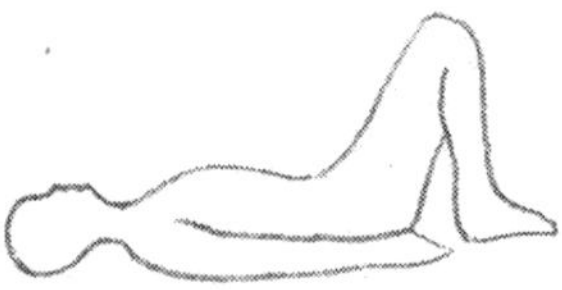

2. Semi-supine – dynamic

Inhale raise arms overhead. Exhale bring back by hips. x4

Inhale raise arms overhead, stay 4 breaths

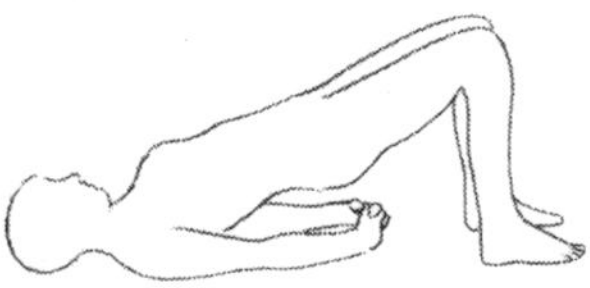

3. Dvipāda Pīṭham – dynamic + static

Inhale lift pelvis and arms, exhale lower x4

Inhale stay 2-6 breaths

Counterpose - Apānāsana

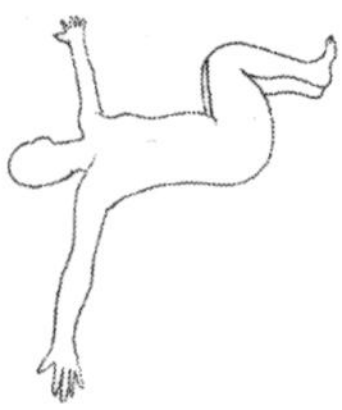

4. Jaṭhara parivṛtti - dynamic

Exhale lower legs half way to floor x2 R + L

Exhale lower legs to floor x2 R + L

Counterpose with Apānāsana

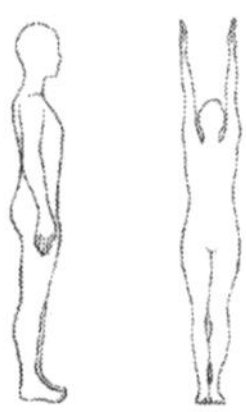

5. Tāḍāsana - dynamic

Inhale raise arms, exhale lower. x4

Static 4 breaths

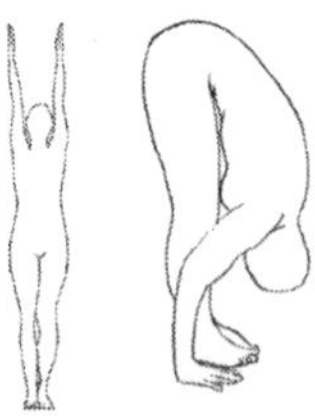

6. Ardha Uttānāsana /Uttānāsana - dynamic

Inhale raise arms, exhale fold forward to 90' arms to low back x4

Inhale raise arms, exhale fold forward x4

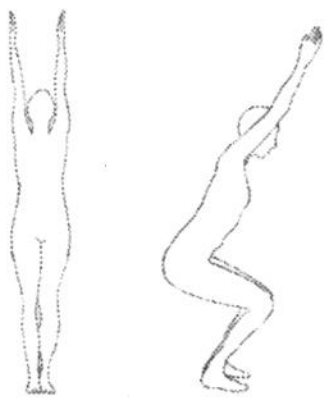

7. Ardha Utkaṭāsana/Utkaṭāsana - dynamic

Inhale raise arms exhale squat half way x4

Inhale raise arms exhale squat full way x4

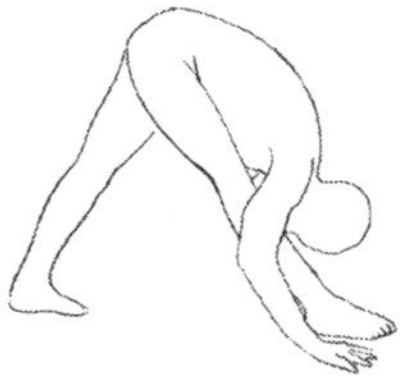

8. Parśva Uttānāsana - static

Inhale raise arms, exhale fold forward over front leg.

Stay 4 breaths R + L

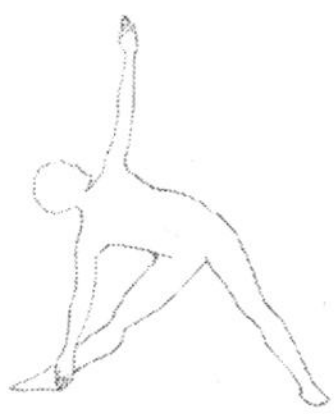

9. Trikoṇāsana - dynamic

Inhale raise arms to shoulder height.

Exhale tilt into posture. R x 4, L x 4.

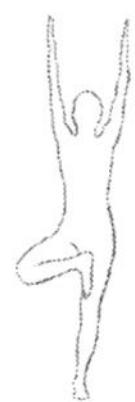

10. Vṛkṣāsana – static

Transfer weight to support leg.
Come into position.

Stay 4-6 breaths R + L.
Samasthiti - stay 4 breaths

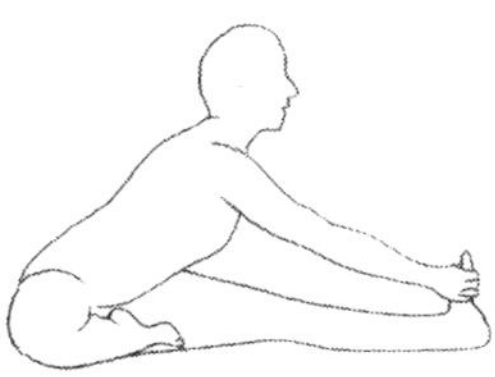

11. Jānuśirṣāsana – static

Inhale raise arms, exhale come into posture.

Stay 4 breaths

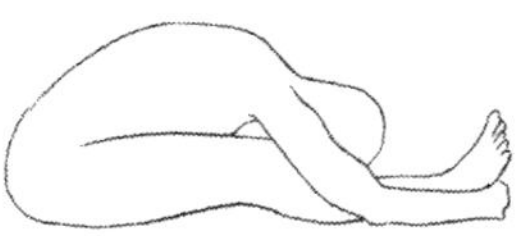

12. Paścimatānāsana – static

Inhale raise arms, exhale come into posture.

Stay 4 breaths. Counterposture apānāsana.

Prāṇāyāma - developing ujjāyī and observe directional flow 8 mins

1.After the final asana, practice ujjāyī breath.

Standing in Samāsthiti:

Inhale through mouth raise arms to Tadāsana. Exhale through mouth, lower the arms. 2 breaths

2. Inhale through mouth raise arms to Tadāsana. Exhale through mouth, begin to lower arms.

When arms are half way down, close mouth. Continue to exhale ujjāyī through throat as arms lower. 4 breaths

3. Sit using supports, (chair, stool, blocks or blankets). Establish uplifted spine, comfortable hips.

R palm on chest. L palm on abdomen: observe inhale at chest, exhale from abdomen. 4 breaths

4. Apply ujjāyī and continue to observe directional flow of breath.
4 breaths

5. Continue ujjāyī, lengthen exhalations within comfortable range.
4 breaths

6. Place hands in Jñāna mudrā. Continue ujjāyī, observing inhale at chest, ex from abdomen. 4 breaths

7. Let the lengthening release. Observe natural breathing. 4 breaths

Dhāranā - concentration 6-8 mins

The focus for this practice is internal cleanliness/purity of the mind.

Have an object ready for concentration practice. Use a white candle flame if this signifies purity for you and if it will engage your attention and feel positive. Or choose something else e.g. a natural object, a religious icon, image of an inspirational person etc.

Come into a comfortable seated position on a chair, blocks or kneeling stool.

Rest the lengthened arms onto the legs, hands in Jñāna mudrā.

Lower the eyes and observe the breath settling into a gentle, regular rhythm. 4 breaths

With each exhale feel that you are letting go of scattered thinking and settling. 4 breaths

Now let your eyes rest on your candle or chosen 'pure' object.

Let your full concentration remain on it as you sit.

If your attention wanders, bring it back and re-focus. 4 mins

Let your attention gradually move back to your breathing. Bring your hands together in your lap.

Let your gaze slowly raise and come out of the practice.

Relaxation 10 mins

Internal Śauca - Cleansing Light Guided Visualisation

Come into a comfortable semi-supine position. Feel the back of the pelvis settling into the mat.

Anchoring the pelvis, lengthen then release the spine.

Let the hands turn gently upwards, palms facing the ceiling. Hands are soft, fingers lightly curled. Let the upper arms rotate softly upwards and outwards, shoulders relax back, chest gently opens.

Let the legs stay bent if you enjoy this support into your back. Or slowly stretch out the right leg and then the left. Let them rest. Allow the heels to release into the mat, toes softly easing outwards.

Feel the centre point at the back of the head resting perfectly. Let the neck relax, head fully supported by the floor.

Enjoy the whole body resting and releasing. If there are any points of discomfort, adjust them gently now.

Begin to visualise yourself lying in a space where you feel restful, undisturbed. It may be a real place or imagined.

The air is warm and still and the surface you are lying on is soft and velvety beneath you.

You feel warm and calm, there is plenty of time. You feel spacious and easy.

As you rest, begin to visualise a gentle white light glowing in the centre of your chest.

Feel the glow brighten as you inhale and dim subtly when you exhale.

As you watch, the glow of light spreads into your whole rib cage and chest, softly pulsating with your breath.

Each time you inhale and the light brightens, feel that the heart and lungs are becoming cleansed and energised. Each time you exhale, feel any impurities in your cardiovascular system release.

Now see the glowing light ease down into your upper and lower abdomen.

Feel the digestive system becoming cleansed and energised as you inhale. Impurities releasing as you exhale.

Feel the warmth of the light travel into your legs and feet. As you inhale your muscles feel energised and nourished, as you exhale muscular tension is released from the lower limbs.

Let the glow of light ease steadily up into your shoulders, arms and hands.

As you inhale the light brightens and your shoulders, arms and hands feel energised and cleansed.

As you exhale strain and stiffness from the upper limbs are released.

The glow of white light eases up into the space between your eyebrows and settles there.

As you inhale the light glows brightly, your thoughts are positive and full of enthusiasm.

As you exhale, the glow softens and stale, negative and unhelpful thought patterns release.

Inhaling your mind feels open and light. Exhaling worries and overwhelm reduce.

Now begin to let the image of the glowing white light fade, leaving you mentally refreshed, renewed and purified.

You rest for a few moments feeling calm, clear and optimistic.

Become more aware of yourself lying in your space and allow your breath to deepen.

Make small movements with fingers and toes and then let the movements grow so that you gradually reawaken yourself in ways that you enjoy.
Rest onto your side for a few breaths before coming up to sitting.

Off the Mat Practices

Slow down. Let thoughts slow down too.

When harassed by doubt, cultivate the opposite attitude – optimism.

Take part in activities which release endorphins. Do what you love.

Go to beautiful places and stare. Spend time in nature.

Hang out with cheerful people. Call someone who makes you laugh. Watch a funny film.

Cultivate simplicity in your life. Do one thing at a time with focus.

Go into a shop with wafting bakery smells – have clarity – don't buy anything.

See something you would like in a shop window or online – have clarity – don't follow up.

When you become aware you are comparing yourself negatively to others – think of all your skills.

Contemplations

I cleanse my mind of negative thoughts, feelings and emotions.

Reducing busyness offers me space for peace.

Purity and simplicity bring ease.

In the stillness of silence, I connect with my essence.

My senses are quiet and I am settled.

I feel light, bright and optimistic.

All is well in my world.

I feel calm and clear.

Observing my breath, I steady myself.

Bhagavad Gītā 17:14: *Calmness, gentleness, silence, self-restraint and purity: these are the disciplines of the mind.*

Take time to reflect

Which negative thought patterns most commonly affect you?

How can you become more aware of them arising?

How can you reduce them?

Which positive thought patterns most commonly affect you?

How can you encourage them?

What will greater mental focus bring you?

Study 3 - Understanding Saṃtoṣa

Sūtra 2:42: saṃtoṣāt-anuttamaḥ sukha-lābhaḥ ||42||

From contentment, unsurpassed happiness is attained.
Paul Harvey

Introduction 5 mins

Sūtra 2:42: saṃtoṣāt-anuttamaḥ sukha-lābhaḥ ||42||

From contentment, unsurpassed happiness is attained.
Paul Harvey

The third lesson of this niyama course is a contemplation on contentment, in Sanskrit 'saṃtoṣa'. Contentment is a state of deep satisfaction, one where we are able to accept things exactly as they are without feeling they should or could be changed. However, contentment in this context is not resignation or passive acceptance of circumstances and unnecessary sufferings. It is having a true understanding of our capabilities and limitations and then allowing plans to grow from an accurate perception of our present reality.

In sūtra 2:42 Patañjali describes saṃtoṣa as 'unsurpassed' or 'supreme' happiness - 'sukha-lābha'. By defining it in this way, he distinguishes it from temporary forms of happiness such as those we experience on special occasions when we are celebrating amongst family and friends. In such moments we feel elated, but after a short while when the celebrations end and family and friends disperse, feelings of happiness transition to something more subdued, perhaps even disappointment and dissatisfaction. The Bhagavad Gītā considers this thought pattern too:

Then those who are established in equanimity... with unswerving discrimination and free from delusion, they never become falsely elated by pleasant experience or depressed by bad.
Bhagavad Gītā 5:19-20

Discontent and dissatisfaction arise when we want things to stay as they are; for the fun of family celebrations not to be followed by a return to work, for warm summer weather not to give way to winter. We become attached to what we enjoy and feel disturbed when it is no longer available. Possessions can create similar thought patterns. A new car for example, previously coveted for its up to date systems and extra features, soon becomes part of the background to the day and simply a means of getting to where we want to go.

The happiness we get from acquiring passions is only temporary. We need to find new ones and acquire them to sustain this sort of happiness. There is no end to it. But true contentment... is in a class by itself.
TKV Desikachar, commentary on 2:42 (The Heart of Yoga p179)

The pleasantness arising from contentment goes much deeper than the transient types of happiness described above. The root of the word saṃtoṣa is 'tuṣ' which means 'to enjoy' (C. Chapple p71). Saṃtoṣa is a deep and sustained sense of enjoyment and satisfaction, unaffected by time and external circumstances. The Sanskrit 'sam' means together. So saṃtoṣa is to 'enjoy-together'. To have a feeling of satisfaction which is the result of being linked to something much deeper and more long term within us – to Atman/Self/essence. Saṃtoṣa is both profound and enduring because it arises from a connection with our essential nature or Self.

Development of saṃtoṣa can be supported through practice of the first niyama śauca and it is useful to consider their relationship. When we make efforts to 'purify' externally - our living spaces, our diet, our sleep routines, our bodies - a sense of ease and space arises. For example, we sweep the winter debris from the patio, pot up some spring flowers and sit next to them with a glass of water. We appreciate the cleared space, enjoy the fresh colours of new growth and things feel good in our world, for a while. We make efforts to 'purify' internally – by interrupting negative thinking, engaging in self-study to recognise misperceptions, reducing unhealthy mental habits and beliefs. We adopt daily yoga practices, do digital-detox, go outside in nature more and we feel clearer, more focussed, for a while.

Although the efforts we make create short-lived changes at first, each 'cleansing' creates supportive latent impressions/habits (saṃskāra) which gradually build towards something more long term. Each mental or physical 'clear space' we create using śauca, results in a moment of pleasantness and optimism – of sattva. We become encouraged and keep on trying. Eventually, sattva can be more present and sustained and this enables us to link with something profound within ourselves. From this connection, a longer term and deeper form of happiness - saṃtoṣa can become established. The process of taking care of what we have, appreciating what we don't need and becoming more aware of where our attachments lie, takes us closer and closer to satisfaction. Śauca is a key tool for development of saṃtoṣa, it supports the mind to have 'fitness for the vision of the Self'. (Chapple translation of PYS 2:41)

Leaving the transient, find joy in the Eternal: Set not your heart on another's possessions.
Īśa Upaniṣat 1

When explaining saṃtoṣa in his book The Dictionary of Yoga (p309), the yoga scholar George Feuerstein cites the Māhabārata which describes the quality of contentment as 'the highest heaven', 'supreme joy'.

'There is nothing higher than satisfaction ('tushtil'). It is complete in itself.'
Māhabārata X11:21.2

We begin this third study by directing our attention to how the breath moves the soft tissue of the pelvic floor. We use Balāsana posture - Child's Pose as it facilitates good observation of pelvic floor movement.

Allow your breathing to be soft, relaxed and spontaneous.

The blank page opposite is available for you to record your observations later.

Come to high kneeling. Slowly and with control, ease your pelvis backwards and down towards your legs. Let the lower spine stretch back as you lower.

Support the head with blocks if helpful. Let the arms be alongside the thighs or stay forwards. Settle.

Bring your attention to your pelvic floor, the area from the pubic bone at the front, to your tailbone at the back and side to side between the sitting bones. Notice any contracting areas, release gently with each exhalation.

Now begin to notice how the pelvic floor moves as you breathe in and out. 6 breaths

What happens on the inhale? What happens on the exhale? Continue to observe.

Notice how these micro movements occur effortlessly, organically, gently, whole body-system working together.

Now contract the pelvic floor in and up. 6 breaths

When the pelvic floor is contracted and held what changes do you notice as you breathe?

Where do you feel the breath? What happens on the inhale? What happens on the exhale?

Now let the pelvic floor gradually release, let your attention come to the forehead where it is resting.

Then bring your hands alongside your shoulders and use your arms to push your back gently up.

Notes on Breath Observations

What did you observe in the pelvic floor on the inhalations?

What did you observe in the pelvic floor on the exhalations?

How did movements change when the pelvic floor was drawn upwards?

On the inhales?

On the exhales?

Saṃtoṣa – contentment

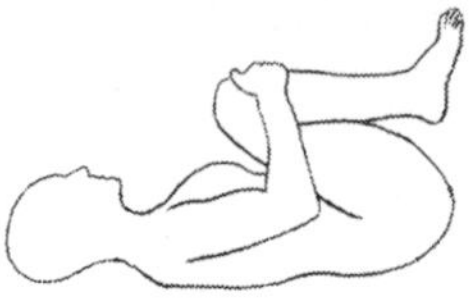

1. Apānāsana - dynamic

Exhale draw knee to chest. Inhale release.

x4 R + L. x4 both legs

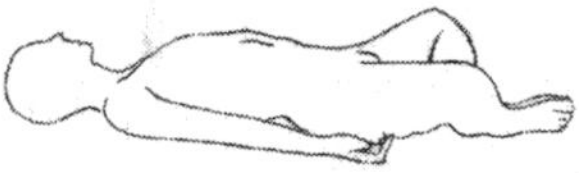

2. Supta baddha koṇāsana – static

Bend knees over chest, part them. Circle clockwise/anticlockwise x4

Static: Lower feet, open knees to floor, stay 4 breaths

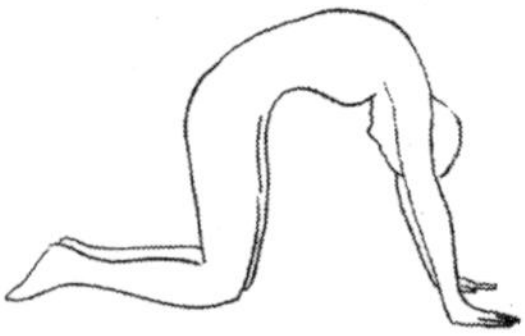

3. Cakravākāsana – dynamic

Inhale squeeze shoulder blades together, open chest

Exhale draw abdomen in and pull pelvis back from gripped fingertips

x4 rounds

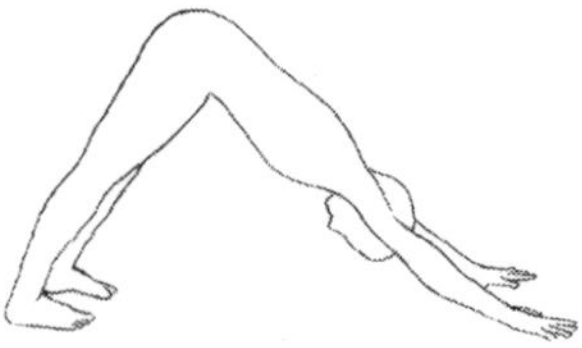

4. Adhomukha svānāsana – static

Come into posture from kneeling

Stay 4-6 breaths

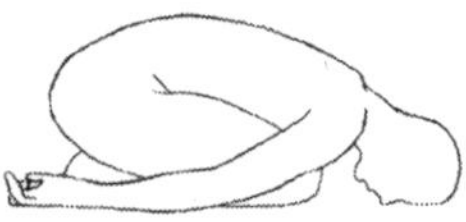

5. Balāsana – static

Stay 4 breaths

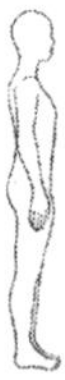

6. Samasthiti – static

Inhale lift sternum and crown, exhale keep lifted

Stay 4-6 breaths

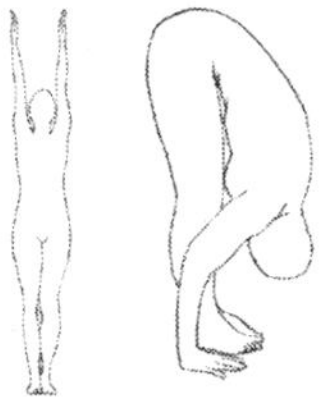

7. Ardha Uttānāsana/Uttānāsana – static

Inhale raise arms, exhale fold forwards to 90° x4

Inhale raise arms, exhale full fold forwards stay 4-6 breaths

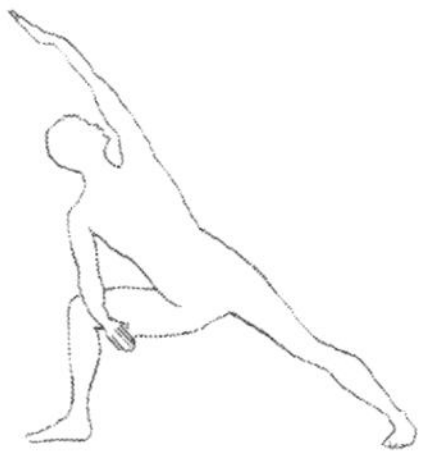

8. Parśva Koṇāsana – static

Inhale raise arms to shoulder height,

exhale lateral flexion, R arm overhead, L arm folds to bent L leg

Stay 4-6 breaths. Repeat to R.

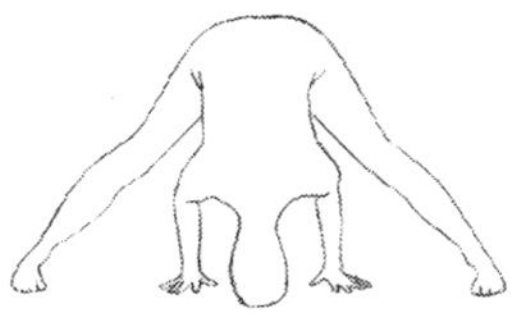

9. Prasārita Pāda Uttānāsana

Inhale raise arms overhead, exhale fold forwards to support/floor.

Stay 4-6 breaths

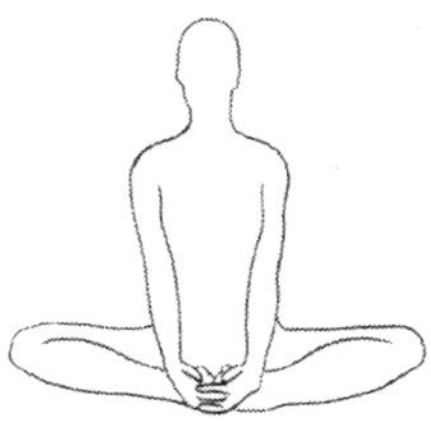

10. Baddha koṇāsana – static

Lift sternum on inhale, keep lifted on exhale.

Stay 4 breaths

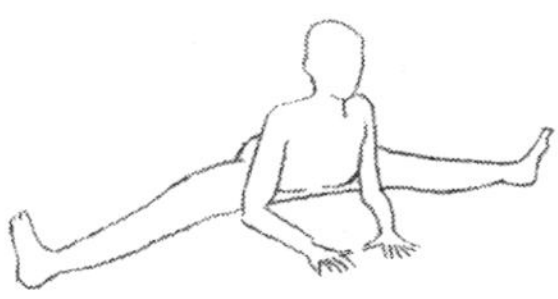

11. Upaviṣṭa koṇāsana – static

Inhale raise arms, exhale fold forwards hands to floor

Stay 4 breaths

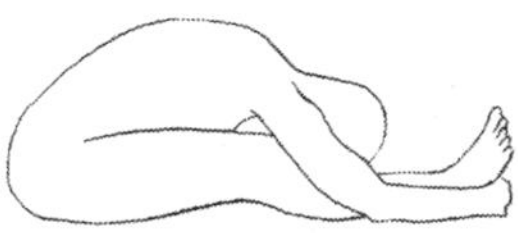

12. Paścimatānāsana - static.

Begin in daṇḍāsana. Inhale raise arms, exhale fold forwards.

Stay 4 breaths

Prāṇāyāma - developing ujjāyī and observe directional flow. 6-8 mins

Sit with support using chair, stool etc. Establish an uplifted spine and comfort in the hips and legs.

1. Revise ujjāyī breathing:

Inhale through mouth raise arms above head. Exhale through mouth, begin to lower arms.

When arms half way down, close mouth. Continue to exhale ujjāyī as arms lower. 4 breaths

2. Continue ujjāyī. R palm on chest, L palm on abdomen - inhale at chest, exhale from abdomen. 6 breaths

3. Place hands in Jñāna mudrā. Continue ujjāyī observing inhale at chest, exhale from abdomen. 6 breaths

4. Continue ujjāyī, lengthening exhalations within own comfortable range. 6 breaths

5. Let the lengthening release. Observe natural breathing. 4 breaths

Dhāraṇā - concentration 6-8 mins

The focus for this practice is the feeling of satisfaction or contentment.

Students choose from a selection of quotations on saṃtoṣa written on slips of paper, ensuring it is meaningful for them, engages their attention and feels positive. Readers will find a selection of quotations listed in the 'contemplations' section at the end of this lesson.

Come into a comfortable seated position. Read the contentment quote several times.

Rest the lengthened arms onto the legs, hands in Jñāna mudrā.

Lower the eyes and observe the breath settling into a gentle, regular rhythm. 4 breaths

Let the eyes come to rest on your phrase or quotation, or if memorised, let the eyes close. 4 mins

Repeat it gently to yourself, perhaps linking it to the flow of the breath.

Let your full concentration remain on the words as you sit.
If your attention wanders, bring it back.

Let your attention gradually move back to your breathing.

Gently bring your hands into your lap, R palm resting on top of L.
Let your eyes slowly re-focus.

Saṃtoṣa - contentment

Let the legs stay in semi-supine position. Feel the back of the pelvis settling into the mat. Anchoring the pelvis, lengthen up through the spine to the crown, then release.

Let the hands turn gently upwards, palms facing the ceiling. Hands soft, fingers lightly curled.

Let the upper arms rotate softly outwards so that the shoulders relax back and the chest opens.

Let the legs stay in supine if this supports your back well. Or slowly stretch out the right leg and then the left. Rest.

Feel that the centre point at the back of the head resting perfectly, neck relaxed. Enjoy the whole body releasing.

Imagine that someone you know and love has experienced a success. Notice the quality of the feelings which arise, perhaps joy, pleasantness, happiness, satisfaction, contentment. How good it feels to wish them well.

Now, begin to recognise some of your own successes. Let them come to mind, large or small. Experience the sensations of achievement, happiness, satisfaction, completion, contentment which they have brought you.

Allow these feelings of contentment and satisfaction to fully develop.

Experience them in the chest and ribcage. Let them deepen and grow with each inhalation.

Now, on each exhalation let this positive glow flow outwards into the shoulders, softly down through arms and be exhaled gently through the hands and fingers. The upper body glowing with pleasantness and contentment.

Let your awareness move deep into the core of the chest, into the heart space. Let feelings of satisfaction and ease develop there. Appreciate aspects of your health which you enjoy and the freedom for practice which they bring.

Let gratitude ease down into the solar plexus. Let contentment with all that you already are soften the solar plexus and bring relaxation. Cultivate contentment in the lower abdominal area.

Feel secure, optimistic and satisfied. Allow these to develop on your inhales and then with your exhales let these positive and pleasant feelings flow softly through the hips, down through the lengths of the legs, through the ankles, through the feet and finally through the toes and away.

Take attention up into the collar bones, throat, neck and vocal chords. Let softness and lightness develop here.

Feel that your voice can lightly express optimism and goodwill.

Let lightness and pleasantness spread up through the neck and softly into the face. Your face is relaxed and your expression is open and optimistic.

Let lightness and pleasantness spread inside the head. Your mind feels soothed, filled with attitudes of compassion, goodwill and delight in the achievements of others.

Let your exhalations flow softly out through the back of the head. The whole head and neck are soft and relaxed.

The whole body rests in contentment and pleasantness. Stay quietly here for a few moments.

Let your breath deepen. Make small movements with fingers and toes and then let the movements grow.

Gradually reawaken yourself in the ways that you enjoy.

When you feel ready, rest onto your side for a few breaths before coming up to sitting.

Off the Mat Practices

Start a gratitude journal. At the end of each day record two good things from that day.

Spend time with your favourite people.

Sit in a room in your home and take time to look around. Appreciate the soft furnishings, objects gathered on travels or gifted from family and friends. Appreciate the comfort, the colours, etc.

Each time you have an 'I need…' thought, interrupt it and list two or three similar things you already have.

Each time you feel discontent - cultivate contentment.

The mind is made restless and dissatisfied by the five kleśa which stir up discontent. Study Yoga Sūtra chapter 2:3-9 where they are explained. Become more alert to them in yourself.

Persevere: *'Saṃtoṣa has bearing on mental activities such as study, on physical efforts and even how we earn our living. Saṃtoṣa is about ourselves, what we have and how we feel about what has been given to us….. Instead of despair when our actions don't yield desired results, we progress and learn from our actions'.*
TKV Desikacher, Religiousness in Yoga p111

Watch your thoughts and try to understand where desires arise from.

Carry a small notebook with you for a week. Note down strong desires when they arise. What do you desire? What circumstances cause more desires to surface? Where/when are you most often content?

Contemplations

'Contentment exists not in great wealth, but in few wants.' Epictetus

In the still depth of my soul I am undisturbed by the surface waves of experience.

Whatever comes of itself I accept, and remain calmly centred within.

Desires don't control my thoughts. Within me lies the source of pure joy and peace.

I live life now in the present moment and remain open to positive changes.

'Joy is not in things, it is in us.' Charles Wagner

How does pratyahara (withdrawal from senses) support saṃtoṣa?
I stay steady within the outgoing senses.

Be still within.

'You will never be able to change things outwardly in such a way as to make them, ever pleasing to you. Therefore, change yourself.'
Paramhansa Yogananda, Autobiography of a Yogi.

My essential nature, Self, is like a lake, its natural state is calm and crystal clear.

I am *'sat cit ānanda'* – pure, blissful awareness.

Silence and stillness bring contentment and peace.

Simple ways of living come easily. I follow the middle path and am balanced and moderate in all things.

'Simple living, high thinking.' Stephen Sturgess, The Yoga Book

Watch your thoughts. Try to understand your desires and discontent.
Observe yourself consistently for a week. Note down strong desires when they arise.
What do you desire?

Which circumstances cause more desires to surface?

Where/when are you most often content?

Is there a desire which you tend towards often which disturbs contentment e.g. travel, money, relationships, property, social status, knowledge?

Is it longstanding? Or are your 'wants' more changeable and short term?

How do you feel when you don't get what you want? Or get what you don't want?

Are you moved a great deal or a little?

Study 4 - Understanding Tapas

Sūtra 43: kāya-indriya-siddhiḥ aśuddhi-kṣayāt-tapasaḥ ||43||

From self-discipline, impurities diminish and accomplishment in the body and senses.
Paul Harvey

Study 4: Understanding Tapas

Introduction 5 mins

Sūtra 43: kāya-indriya-siddhiḥ aśuddhi-kṣayāt-tapasaḥ ||43||

From self-discipline, impurities diminish and accomplishment in the body and senses.
Paul Harvey

Tapas is the third niyama within Patañjali's eight limb yoga system. The word 'tapas' comes from the root 'tap' which means to heat or cleanse. Tapas is self-purification. It consists of the efforts we make to remove impurities in the body, mind and behaviour. It is also the ability to continue with our efforts towards self-purification, even when they bring discomfort. The heat of tapas is positive and necessary for change.

'Tapas involves observing disciplines which challenge us and thereby generate 'heat'. This heat is like the fuel of change and transformation, giving us vitality and the strength to pursue our goals'.
Ranju Roy and Dave Charlton, Embodying the Yoga Sūtra, p241

At times, tapas has been defined as penance, dietary austerity even mortification. But tapas within the yoga system is not extreme austerities or discipline for the sake of discipline. It is reducing and eventually removing anything which hinders the healthy functioning of the body, mind and the eleven sense organs (see sūtra 2:18). We approach the practice of tapas with the qualities of ahiṃsā, being thoughtfully disciplined about food, sleep, exercise, work, speech and time for self-reflection.

'...any means of tapas we use must do us good. Simply to fast for twenty days without reason could cause us great difficulties. If by austerity we mean austerity with reason, it is tapas. Tapas must not make us suffer. This is very important.'
TKV Desikachar, Religiousness in Yoga, p113

The overarching purpose of tapas is to cultivate the conditions where sattva can be present. Through disciplined and sustained practice of yama, niyama, āsana, prāṇāyāma, pratyahara and dhāraṇā we cultivate in the body and mind the qualities of balance, stability, lightness and clarity.

Bhagavad Gītā 6:10-12

The yogin should concentrate constantly….
Establishing a firm seat for himself in a clean place…
There, having directed his mind to a single object,
With his thought and the activity of the senses controlled,
Seating himself on the seat, he should practice
Yoga for the purpose of self-purification'.

Winthrop Sargeant translation.

Through a disciplined approach to yoga practices we manage the quality, quantity and direction of our energies. Then practice, supported by healthy lifestyle choices, helps us to become disentangled from unhelpful habits and attachments:

Bhagavad Gītā 6:17

For him who is moderate in food and diversion,
Whose actions are disciplined,
Who is moderate in sleep and waking,
Yoga destroys all sorrow.

Winthrop Sargeant translation

Our ability to influence the guṇa through purifying diet is emphasised by the teachings of TKV Desikachar:

'Your mind is a product of your food. Memory is linked to food. My stability, my confidence, is linked to food. All these facts are mentioned in the texts. For these reasons I said that food is very important and becomes me. Not just the muscles, but the whole of me, the whole personality'. Interview in the journal Viniyoga Italia on 'Yoga and Wellbeing'

This is indeed mentioned in the texts – one example is in 17:8-10 of the Bhagavad Gītā:

'Men who are pure like food which is pure: which gives health, mental power, strength and long life; which has taste, is soothing and nourishing, and which makes glad the heart of man.

Men of Rajas like food of Rajas: acid and sharp, and salty and dry, and which brings heaviness and sickness and pain.

Men of darkness eat food which is stale and tasteless, which is rotten and left overnight, impure, unfit for holy offerings'.

TKV Desikachar succinctly expressed tapas in relation to food during a class on Sāṃkhya in 1979: *'As is the food in front of you, so is the mind behind you.'*

Source: yogastudies.org/sanskrit/annam

Śri T Krishnamacharya taught that moderation of food is accompanied by moderation of speech as components of tapas. The latter is evidenced in the Bhagavad Gītā 17:15:

'Words which give peace, words which are good and beautiful and true, and also the reading of sacred books; this is the harmony of words.'

A disciplined approach, incorporating good food, sleep and communication, together with regular yoga practice, support sattva within our systems. Healthfulness and steadiness become established, leading to mental clarity and sustained awareness. Bhagavad Gītā 6:18-19:

When the mind of a yogi is in harmony and finds rest in the Spirit within, all restless desires gone, then he is a Yukta, one in God.

Then his soul is a lamp whose light is steady, for it burns in a shelter where no winds come.

Chapter 17 translations - Juan Mascaro

Take time to reflect

Reflect upon and record any personal responses to the teachings on tapas…

Record any experiences you feel are relevant to the practice of self-purification…

Which do you find difficult/easier?

Moderation in sleep?

Moderation with food?

Moderation in speech?

Listening attentively?

Note any questions which you could investigate which might bring clarification….

The purpose of this first practice is to direct your attention towards your body and breath. In previous lessons we observed how the breath moves the soft tissue in the abdomen, pelvic floor and the bones of the pelvic basin. In this lesson we explore how the breath moves the spinal column.

After this practice, you might like to make notes on your observations. Allow your breathing to be soft, relaxed, unrestricted and spontaneous, preferably through the nostrils, but if this is uncomfortable, through the mouth.

Come into a balanced semi-supine position. Right side and left sides of the body equally resting.

Feel the back of the pelvis settling into the mat. Bring your attention to the sacrum and to the tailbone.

Can you feel the lower back gently lift slightly as you inhale and release down as you exhale?

Watch how this subtle rocking motion links with the phases of the breath.

Observe how your lumbar spine also follows this movement pattern, arching up slightly on the in breath and lowering down on the out breath.

Let your attention ease up through the spine and continue your observation of how each part of the spinal column moves with the breath.

Observe the thoracic spine.

Observe the cervical spine.

Where do you notice free movement? Where is it more limited?

Can you explore, through observation, where any limitations originate?

Allow your attention to rise up to the uppermost point of the spine at the skull and then let your attention ease into the space between the eyebrows and settle there.

Notes on Breath Observations

How did you experience the breath movements in each part of the spine?

Lumbar spine?

Thoracic spine?

Cervical spine?

Any areas of limitation?

Could you sense where the limitations originate?

Tapas: self-purification

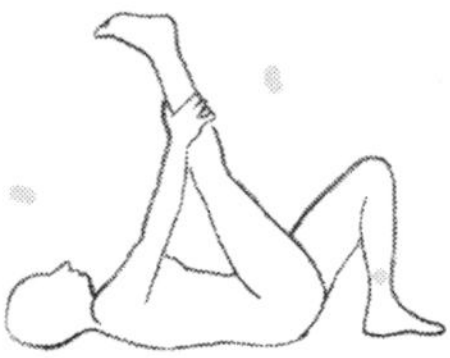

1. Supta pādāṅguṣṭāsana - static

Exhale knee over chest, inhale extend leg, hold with hand

Stay 4-6 breaths R + L

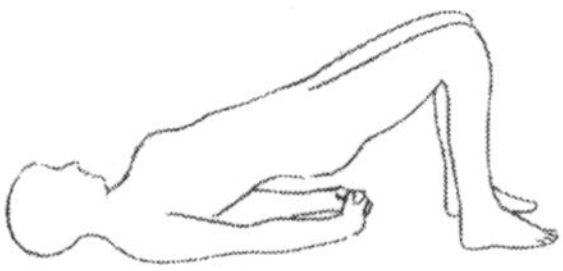

2. Dvipāda Pīṭham - dynamic

Inhale lift pelvis, exhale lower. Arms still. x4

Inhale lift pelvis and arms, exhale lower x4

Static: stay lifted 2-4 breaths

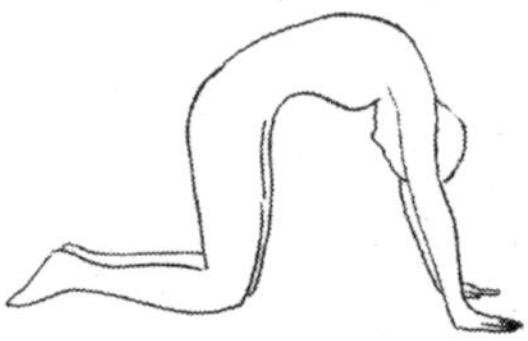

3. Cakravākāsana - dynamic

Inhale squeeze shoulder blades together, open chest

Exhale draw abdomen in and pull pelvis back from gripped fingertips

x4 rounds

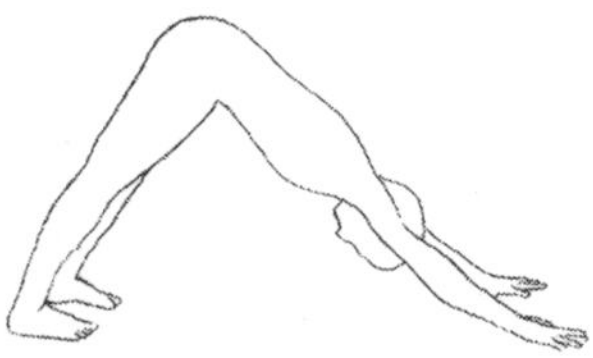

4. Adhomukha svānāsana - static

From all fours exhale lift hips up and back

Inhale wide into chest, exhale from lower abdomen.

Stay 4-6 breaths, repeat

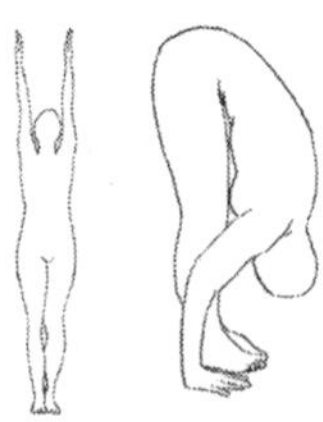

5. Ardha Uttānāsana/Uttānāsana - dynamic

Inhale raise arms, exhale fold forwards to 90° x4

Inhale raise arms, exhale full fold forwards x4

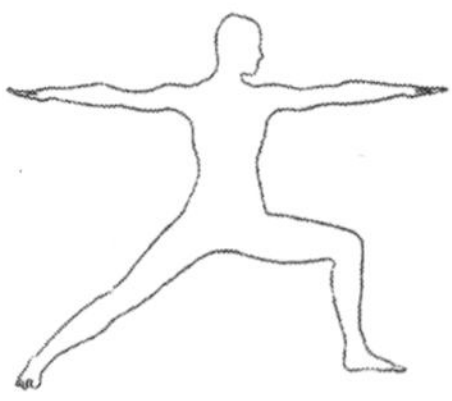

6. Virabhadrāsana – dynamic + static

Inhale sweep arms up bend front knee, exhale release x4

Stay 4 breaths R + L

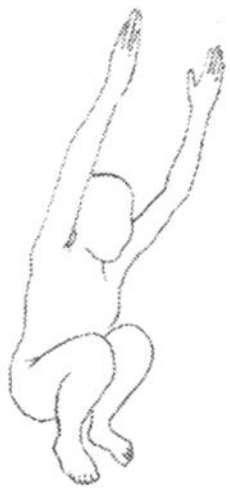

7. Ardha Utkaṭāsana/Utkaṭāsana - dynamic

Inhale raise arms. exhale bend knees into half squat x4

Repeat full squat x4

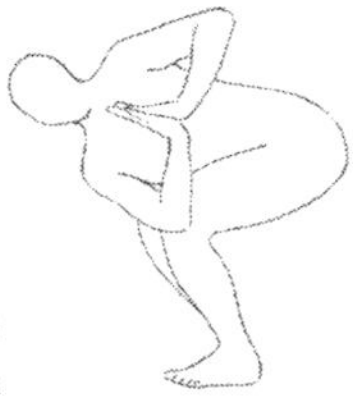

8. Parivṛtti Utkaṭāsana – static

Inhale raise arms, exhale bend knees, twist to right. Stay 4 breaths

Repeat L

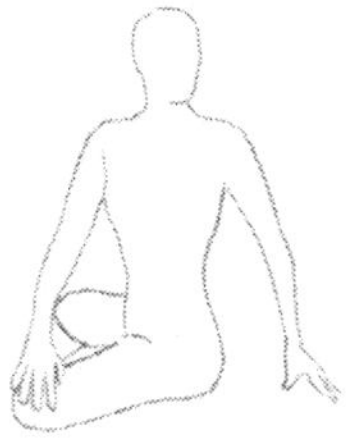

9. Parivṛtti Sukhāsana – dynamic

Inhale twist to R, rotating gradually 4 breaths

Repeat L

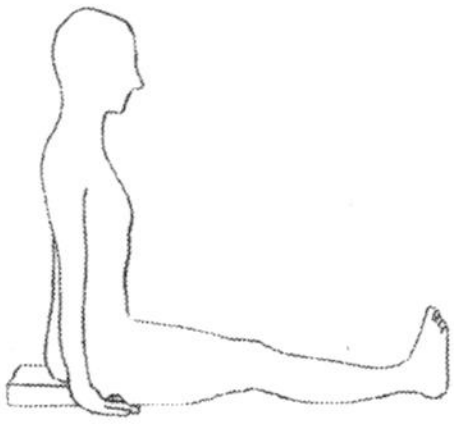

10. Daṇḍāsana – dynamic

Inhale raise arms, exhale lower,
keep sternum lifting x4

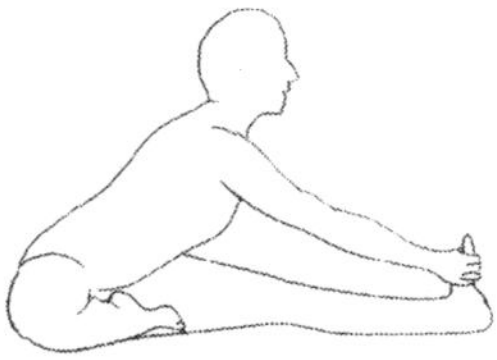

11. Jānuśirṣāsana – dynamic

Inhale raise arms, exhale fold forwards, x4 R+L

Repeat R + L

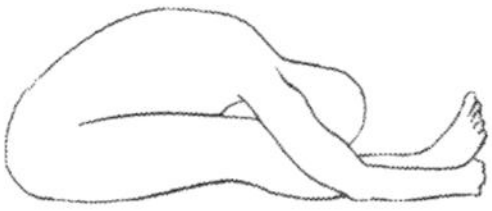

12. Paścimatānāsana – dynamic

Inhale raise arms, exhale fold forwards, x4

Prānāyāma - ujjāyī and breath direction 6-8 mins

Sit comfortably with support. Establish an uplifted spine and comfort in the hips and legs.

1. Revise ujjāyī breathing: 4 breaths

Inhale through mouth raise arms above head. Exhale through mouth, lower arms for length of exhalation.

When arms half way down, close mouth. Continue to exhale ujjāyī as arms lower.

2. Continue ujjāyī. R palm on chest, L palm on abdomen - inhale at chest, exhale from abdomen. 6 breaths

3. Place hands in Jñāna mudrā. Continue ujjāyī and observing - in at chest, ex from abdomen. 8 breaths

4. Continue ujjāyī, lengthening exhalations within own comfortable range. 6 breaths

5. Return to simple breathing. 4 breaths

Dhāranā - concentration 6-8 mins

The focus of this practice is tapas – making efforts to establish healthful habits.

Come to a comfortable seated position. Use any props you need for support.

Let the spine feel long and lifted, shoulders relaxed.

Rest the lengthened arms onto the legs, hands in Jñāna mudrā.

Be aware of your sitting bones grounded into the surface you are sitting on.

Recall that tapas, is self-purification and the ability to stay steady with your efforts.

Focus on the quality of 'sthira' – steadiness and feel established in healthful habits. 1 min

Now let your attention focus on the quality of 'sthiti' – the ability to remain. 1 min

Become focussed on one of these, the one which feels most relevant at this time. 4 mins

Let your full concentration remain on this quality. If your attention wanders, bring it back.

Let your attention gradually move back to your breathing. 1 min

Bring your hands together in the lap. Gradually release your focus and lift your gaze.

Relaxation 10 mins

Relaxation – tapas - nourishing food and heat.

Bring the body into a well-balanced, even position, supine, semi supine or seated if better.

Support any parts of the body that would be more comfortable with blankets, cushions or blocks.

Allow the eyes to close gently, feel that the body is settling and you are in a mood to relax.

Begin to visualise yourself cosily at home on a frosty January morning. Picture yourself sitting in your warm kitchen.

So far on this day, you have completed your personal yoga practice, visited your local grocer and spent the rest of the morning steadily chopping vegetables and making your favourite winter soup.

You are hungry for it now and carefully set the table with your favourite bowl and spoon.

See yourself cut a slice of fresh bread to go with the soup if you wish.

Observe the steaming soup as you pour it into the bowl and sprinkle it with fresh herbs.

Notice the freshness of the colour. Notice the consistency.

You begin to eat, feeling the warm soup on your tongue and enjoying the flavours.

Chewing the fresh bread slowly, you appreciate the soft textures and the creamy butter.

You swallow the soup and feel it pass down into your stomach where it settles. Warm and comforting.

See your body drawing nutrients and energy expertly from it as you eat. Feel the vitamins and minerals being released into the bloodstream and nourishing your muscles, bones, skin and organs.

See the energy from the food being absorbed for growth and repair. Watch as fibre is used to support digestion.

The whole body is nourished by this simple meal and glowing with health, vitality and purpose.

Feel the whole body cared for through your efforts to nourish it with good food.

Your meal is finished now. You feel satisfied, warm and content.

Let yourself rest in this warm, healthfulness for a few moments.

Now begin to let this visualisation gradually release.
Become more aware of yourself resting.

Let your breath deepen. Begin to make small movements which gradually increase.

When you feel ready, roll onto your side and rest there for a moment before gradually coming up to sitting. Take time. No rush.

Off the Mat Practices

Any means of tapas must do us good – be careful to undertake disciplines with good reason.

Take care with how you speak – avoid careless criticisms, gossip and harmful words. Listen attentively and patiently.

Eat foods as fresh and close to their original form as possible, in moderate amounts.

Reduce intake of tea, coffee, alcohol cigarettes, drugs etc.

Don't allow desires to control your actions e.g. don't respond to every hunger pang.

Establish a consistent sleep routine.

Contemplations

I observe my habits and patterns.

I am releasing old behaviours which no longer serve me.

I am steady and clear.

I eat in ways that nourish me.

My daily yoga practice is becoming established.

I enjoy a walk in the light every day.

'*Out of moderation a pure happiness springs.*' Johan Wolfgang van Goethe

Take rest; a field that has rested gives a bountiful crop. Ovid

'*Every failure is a step to success*'. William Whewell

'*Concentrate all your thoughts upon the work at hand. The sun's rays do not burn until brought to a focus*'. Alexander Graham Bell.

Take time to reflect

In which ways is my daily life well balanced? Do I get enough time for thought, leisure, eating, exercise, sleep?

Am I maintaining a regular yoga practice? If not, what is getting in my way?

How can I change things to support myself to practice regularly?

How does reducing impurities in my lifestyle help me to make progress with yoga?

Can I speak gently at all times? How can I avoid being drawn into criticism and gossip?

Am I enjoying a healthful diet which suits my constitution?
How could I improve what I consume?

Study 5 - Understanding Svādhyāya

Sūtra 2:44: svādhyāyāt-iṣṭa-devatā-saṃprayogaḥ ||44||

Study, when it is developed to the highest degree, brings one close to higher forces that promote understanding of the most complex.
TKV Desikachar

Study 5 - Understanding Svādhyāya 75 mins practice

Introduction 5 mins

Sūtra 2:44: svādhyāyāt-iṣṭa-devatā-saṃprayogaḥ ||44||

Study, when it is developed to the highest degree, brings one close to higher forces that promote understanding of the most complex. TKV Desikachar

This lesson focusses on the fourth niyama - svādhyāya. According to TKV Desikachar, 'sva' means self or pertaining to self and ādhyāya means 'to go near', (Religiousness in Yoga p112). Svādhyāya is 'to go near yourself'. Through study, practice and self-enquiry, we try to understand more about ourselves. When we work efficiently with our skills and strengths and reduce our weaknesses, there is 'no limit to our understanding', TKV Desikachar Heart of Yoga p180. Svādhyāya is not simply a process of study, it also encompasses how we apply the things we learn. Students of yoga are required to 'walk the talk'.

There are several techniques available within the yoga system which support self-enquiry. These enquiries are acknowledged to be in-depth and long term for most students and it is recommended that we start where we are:

'Before I enquire into who am I, I must first look at who I am'.
TKV Desikachar, commentary on Bhagavad Gītā 6:20.

It is usual for enquiries to begin at the material level with the body and movements of mind. For example, through the practice of āsana we can observe the condition of our physical bodies. We come to know how it moves, what our habitual movement patterns are, the degree of strength and mobility we have, the location and nature of particular limitations. We expose aspects which might benefit from appropriate treatments or additional care. By observing our breath in āsana we come to understand the relationship between our breath and movement and how using the breath in specific ways can support health. Through prāṇāyāma we become sensitive to our energetic states and how we can positively impact our nervous system by using individualised techniques to bring about sympathetic/parasympathetic regulation. The practices of āsana and prāṇāyāma together with dhāraṇā (concentration) and dhyāna (meditation), bring us closer to an awareness of the movements of our minds, of our moods and our habitual thought patterns. Through sustained practice, over a long period, we reveal the nature of psycho- social influences and cultural conditionings which shape how we present within our communities. As TKV Desikachar said, we do not have a mirror to reflect the qualities of our minds as we do for our physical bodies. Instead yoga offers us the study of profound texts, mantra and chanting, as tools for reflection.

Students of yoga are encouraged to read ancient texts not only for the profound wisdom within them but because such texts provide external references upon which we can structure self-enquiry. By reading, discussing, reflecting and observing our responses to texts such as Patañjali's Yoga Sūtra, the Bible, the Mahābārata and the Qur'an, we illuminate something of ourselves. In this way we are supported to explore where we are, what we are and how we can relate well in our world.

It is not enough to keep ourselves fit. We should know who we are and how we relate to others. TKV Desikachar, Religiousness in Yoga p11.

The repetition of mantra and chanting are also tools for self-enquiry within the yoga system. There are many ways of working with them, here we will consider three ways of using them within our practice. The first, recitation for learning, is exemplified in the traditional way of studying Patañjali's Yoga Sūtra. This method involves learning to recite the whole text by heart, before beginning to discuss the meaning of each individual sūtra with a teacher. The purpose of recitation in the practice of Vēdic chanting is not to dissect and analyse but 'lift up' a student's awareness in order for them to link with something higher. The third approach is when a teacher, who knows us well, gives us a mantra for personal study and practice. All three approaches to chanting support self-enquiry, but in different ways according to their purpose.

'*We cannot simply sit and reflect upon ourselves. We need some external guidance.... Sometimes* svādhyāya *is taken to mean the repetition of specific mantras. If we have a guru who knows us very well, our strengths and weaknesses and interests, he might give us a mantra. When we repeat that mantra, we come into 'contact' with the qualities of our guru; we look at his way of life, how he solves problems, etc. so that we receive guidance'.*
TKV Desikachar, Religiousness in Yoga p112

Self-enquiry using special texts, chanting for understanding and contemplation, developing understanding of yoga with a teacher and studying the lifestyles of accomplished figures, are the techniques of svādhyāya. Svādhyāya is:

'to look at that which helps me understand'.
Paul Harvey

So far in this course we have observed how the breath moves the soft tissue and bony tissue in the pelvis and spine. In this lesson we explore how the breath moves the hips and thigh bones. After the practice, you might like to make notes on the movements you observe. Allow your breathing to be soft, relaxed, unrestricted and spontaneous. Preferably through the nostrils.

Come into semi-supine position. Feel balanced, right side and left side of the body resting equally.

Feel the back of the pelvis settling into the mat.

Let your palms spread on the outsides of your upper thighs/pelvis.

Can you feel how your body widens on the inhalation? How it retracts as you exhale?

Don't try to make the movement happen or become bigger – just observe the degree of movement occurring naturally. 6 breaths

Now let the palms of the hands rest lightly on the fronts of the hip joints. 6 breaths

Observe the breath-movements closely and steadily.
Do you notice any micro-movements here?

Let your attention be released from the hips.

How did you experience the movements at the sides of the thighs and pelvis?

On the inhalations?

On the exhalations?

How did you experience the movements at the front of the hips?

On the inhalations?

On the exhalations?

Svādhyāya: self-study

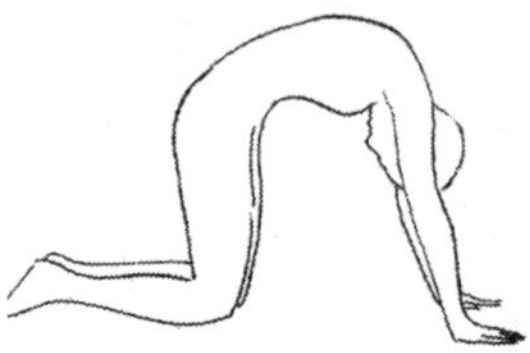

1. Cakravākāsana - dynamic

Inhale squeeze shoulder blades together, open chest

Exhale draw abdomen in and pull pelvis back from gripped fingertips

x4 rounds

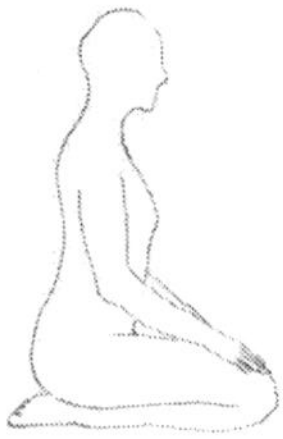

2. Vajrāsana - dynamic

In high kneeling, inhale raise arms, exhale fold forwards arms sweep behind pelvis x4
Rest in Balāsana

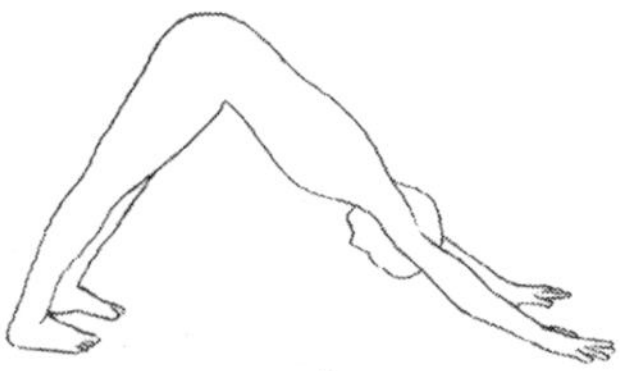

3. Adhomukha svānāsana - static

Inhale on all fours, exhale lift hips up and back

Inhale wide into chest, exhale from lower abdomen.

Stay 4-6 breaths, repeat

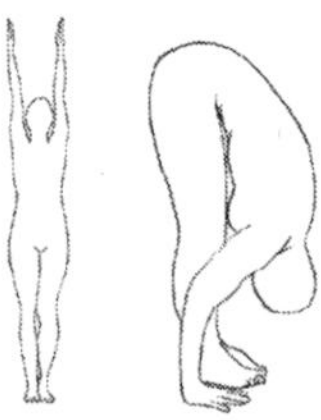

4. Ardha Uttānāsana/Uttānāsana - dynamic

Inhale raise arms, exhale fold forwards to 90' x4

Inhale raise arms, exhale full fold forwards x4

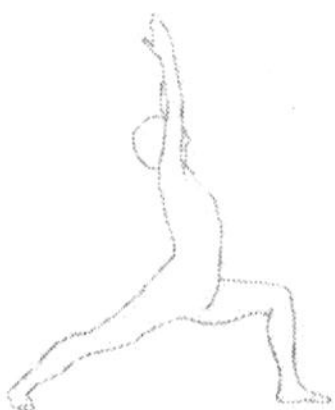

5. Virabhadrāsana - dynamic + static

Inhale sweep arms up bend front knee, exhale release x4

Stay 4 breaths R + L

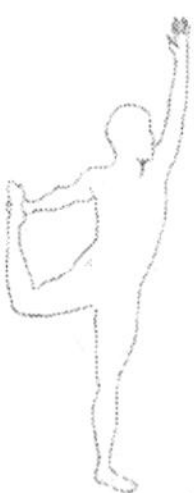

6. Naṭarājāsana - static

Using a belt/wall as supports if needed, come into the pose.

Stay 4-6 breaths R + L

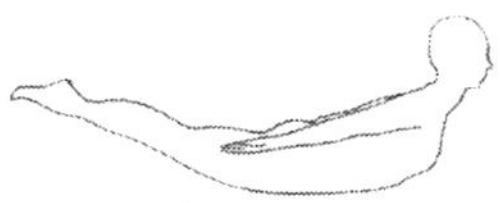

7. Śalabhāsana - dynamic + static

Inhale raise chest and legs, exhale lower x4

Lift and stay 2-4 breaths

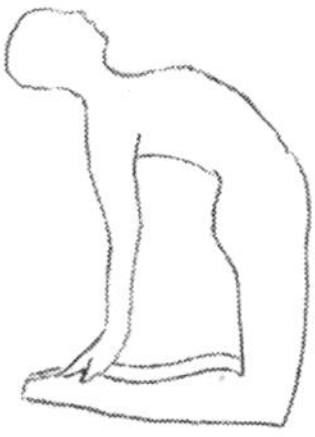

8. Uṣṭrāsana - static

From kneeling, inhale lift chest and pelvis up into posture, stay 2-4 breaths.

Use blocks/chair as supports.

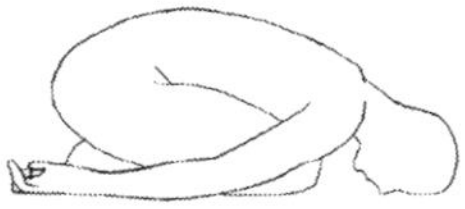

9. Balāsana – static

Stay 4 breaths

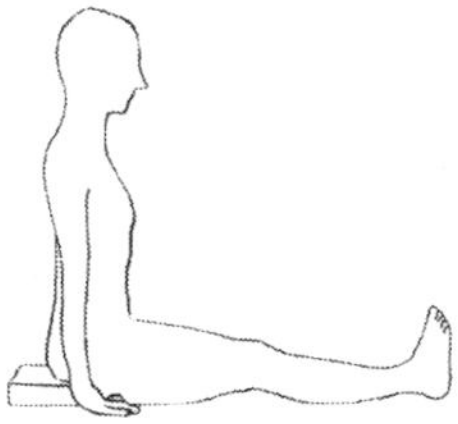

10. Daṇḍāsana – dynamic

Inhale raise arms, exhale lower x4

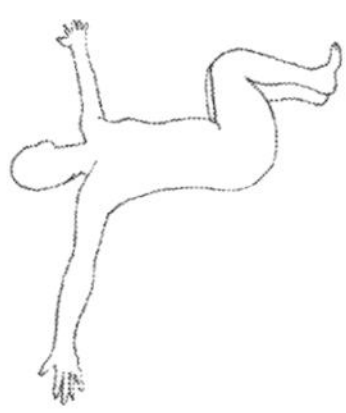

11. Jaṭhara parivṛtti - dynamic

On exhales, lower knees R + L x4

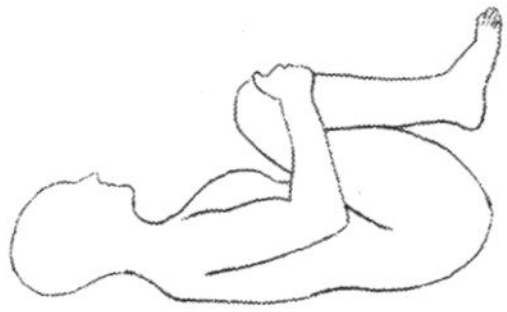

12. Apānāsana - dynamic

Exhale draw knees into chest, inhale release away x4

Prāṇāyāma - ujjāyī using a breath counting technique 6-8mins

1.Come into a comfortable seated position.

2. Teach breath counting technique using left hand.

3. Place R hand in Jñāna mudrā, left thumb ready at base of left forefinger to count.

Establish ujjāyī breathing. 4 breaths

4. Using ujjāyī breathing practice counting. 8 breaths

Check all ok.

5. Continue ujjāyī, using breath counting technique.
Aware of using directional flow as above. 12 breaths

Let exhalations lengthen within own comfortable range.

6. Release ujjāyī and lengthening exhalations.
Simple breath observation. 4 breaths

The focus for this practice is self-understanding.

Come into a comfortable seated position.

Rest the lengthened arms onto the legs, hands in Jñāna mudrā.

Yoga teaches that our true nature, our Essence, or Self, is sat cit ānanda, pure awareness and bliss.

Na ma ma means 'I am not that'. We use awareness of what we are not, as a basis for concentration.

Gather your attention onto your breathing and on each exhalation repeat silently to yourself:

I am not just my physical body. 2 mins

I am not my distracted senses.

I am not my changing moods.

I am not my constantly changing thoughts.

I am not my intellect.

I am not my ego.

I am more than all these.

I am sat (real, true) cit (awareness) ānanda (joy, bliss).

I am pure, blissful awareness.

Choose one of these statements to focus on. 3/4 mins

Hold your attention on this statement. If it wanders, gently bring it back.

Now, let your attention gradually move back to your breathing. 1 min

Bring your hands together in the lap. Gradually release your focus and lift your gaze.

Svādhyāya is self-study, self-reflection, including through special texts.

What has your study of special texts illuminated during self-study? Allow one teaching/phrase/quotation from a text you value to come to mind. It may be from the Yoga Sūtra, the Bible, Bhagavad Gītā, Qur'an. It may be a line of poetry or a quotation from a teacher you respect.

Take a moment and let the core meaning of the teaching come back to you now. Let it distil into a succinct phrase, for example 'My essence is awareness and peace.' Hold this in your heart space and let it settle.

We relax by taking our attention to particular points on the body and repeating the affirmation as we exhale three or four times at each point.

Take the attention first to the feet.

Breathing at the feet – mentally repeat your phrase, e.g. 'I am peaceful', three or four breaths.

Breathing at the legs – mentally repeat your phrase…

Within the abdomen…

Within the solar plexus…

Within the chest…

At the notch of the collar bones…

At the space between the eyebrows…

At the crown of the head…

Now let the attention rest at the sternum.

Breathe and allow your phrase to remain within the heart space. Stay approximately six breaths.

Softly begin to let the phrase fade and allow your attention to drift away from the heart space.

Let the feelings of relaxation stay with you as you begin to become more aware of yourself resting.

Let your breath deepen. Make small movements with fingers and toes and then let the movements grow.

Gradually reawaken yourself in ways that you enjoy.

Rest onto your side for a few breaths before coming up to sitting.

Off the Mat Practices

Be alert when you describe yourself to others. Notice what you say.

Listen carefully when you say: I am… I always… I should be… Is what you say informed by the present? Or is it a habitual portrait?

Use a journal to note down the significant steps forward/developments you have made over recent years.

Write an up to date, short 'bio' to use in new introductions. Keep it factual. Without being boastful, include the aspects of your life which you have made progress with in recent months/years.

For a month observe and record your habits with eating, digestion, sleeping, exercise and activities you find nourishing. What patterns do you notice? Which are helpful? Which are unhelpful?

Choose one unhelpful pattern and plan simple, achievable changes.

Contemplations

I live life with growing awareness.

I look and listen attentively.

I observe my thoughts, feelings, motives and desires.

Samāhita Citta is a firmly rooted steady mind – it describes the qualities of the mind Patañjali considers in Chapter 1 of the Yoga Sūtra.
Consider: 'Am I firmly rooted in my practice?'

Take time to reflect

Consider the changes you have observed in yourself since you began practising yoga…

Make notes on one or two of the most significant ones here….

How are these changes supporting you?

Take a moment to imagine you are peacefully in the closing phase of your life and looking back…

Which activities are you happy to have spent your time and energies on?

Which actions have been worthwhile?

Study 6 – Understanding Īśvara-Pranidhānā

Sūtra 2:45: samādhi-siddhiḥ īśvara-praṇidhānāt

From dedication to the lord, accomplishment in integration.
Paul Harvey

Study 6 - Understanding Īśvara Pranidhānā

2:45. samādhi-siddhiḥ īśvara-praṇidhānāt ||45||

Contemplation and its powers are attained through worship of God.
Bernard Bouanchaud

Perfection in samadhi (arises) from dedication to Īśvara.
Christopher Chapple

Reverence to God promotes the ability to completely understand any object of choice.
TKV Desikachar

Introduction 5 mins

The fifth and final niyama is Īśvara Praṇidhānā. Often translated as 'surrender to the Lord/God'. For yoga practitioners who have a particular faith, this sūtra is quite straightforward. Īśvara Praṇidhānā can be 'surrender' to the supreme being within their faith. But how are we to relate to this sūtra if we are agnostic or atheist or unsure? It can seem difficult to understand the relevance of this sūtra or how it might become part of our practice. Īśvara Praṇidhānā is a teaching which draws many questions and so readers might find it helpful to extend this final phase of the course over a longer period, perhaps repeating the lesson several times. In doing so we can take time to carefully contemplate Īśvara Praṇidhānā within each of the three sūtra where it arises and to explore it from several viewpoints.

It is useful before looking at these three sūtra, to establish that a belief in an omniscient, creator god is not a requirement of yoga. Īśvara appears first in sūtra 1:23:

Īśvara-Praṇidhānā-va
Or surrender to Īśvara

Here Patañjali uses the word 'va'. A small, but highly significant word meaning 'or'. By incorporating it, the teaching of surrender to Īśvara is presented as optional. Patañjali skilfully establishes inclusivity, ensuring that the riches of yoga remain accessible to all. It is also essential for students of yoga to appreciate that the yoga system is separate from the Hindu religion. TKV Desikachar, son and student of Sri T Krishnamacharya, felt that the latter was one of the biggest misunderstandings to have arisen around the teaching and practice of yoga. He took careful steps not to wear religious markings or have religious symbols or objects within teaching spaces, which might make a student feel that the practices of yoga were not for them. Desikachar believed that the teachings of yoga are accessible to everyone, regardless of religion, gender identity, race or age. 'We don't have to accept a notion of God to understand yoga'. (Religiousness in Yoga p33)

Christopher Chapple is a well-respected Sanskrit and sūtra scholar. His translation of sūtra 1:23 is more nuanced than 'surrender to the lord'. Chapple presents the roots of the word Īśvara as 'īś' (command, rule) and 'vṛ' (valuable, eminent, choicest). He records Īśvara as 'master, Lord, king, able to do, capable'. Explaining praṇidhānā as 'dedication, attention paid to, respectful conduct'. It appears here that Īśvara praṇidhānā can be, but need not exclusively be interpreted as 'surrender to God'. It might also be a respectful acknowledgement of our place within the greater system and an awareness of higher qualities which we can link with. With this in mind we can begin to look at each instance that Īśvara praṇidhānāna occurs within Patañjali's Yoga Sūtra.

In sūtra 2:1 Īśvara Praṇidhānā is presented as the third element of kriya yoga:

tapaḥ svādhyāya-īśvara-praṇidhānāni kriyā-yogaḥ

The activities of Yoga are self-discipline, self-study and dedication to the lord.
Paul Harvey

Here, Īśvara Praṇidhānā might be explained as understanding the value of acceptance. We develop habits which support self-discipline, engage in study and self-reflection which shed further light on the quality of our actions and see where these take us. We perform our duties at work, for family and for friends, without feeling the need to control the outcomes. As TKV Desikachar explains, since we can never be sure of the fruits of our actions, it is better to *'remain a little detached and pay more attention to the quality of the actions themselves'*. (Religiousness in Yoga p11). By focussing on the process rather than the goal we are able to avoid disappointments. We become steadier by not being attached. Through the practice of Īśvara Praṇidhānā within the context of kriyā yoga, we discover how surrender supports stability. As such it can form an entry point to understanding Īśvara Praṇidhānā.

Īśvara Praṇidhānā presented as the fifth niyama, (2:32) appears to go much deeper. If we wish to follow the path of yoga it requires greater effort, commitment and self-reflection. Within the context of the niyama, TKV Desikachar teaches Īśvara Praṇidhānā is '*to leave all our actions at the feet of the Lord'*. We make efforts with practice on and off the mat and then, when we have done our best, we leave the fruits of our actions '*in the hands of something higher than ourselves'*. (Religiousness in Yoga p 113). Desikachar offers a further translation of praṇidhānā as 'prostration'. Use of this term implies that we not only 'place down'/submit the fruits of our efforts to something higher, but that we also 'make ourselves low'. In other words, we remain awake to our individual place within a far bigger system. By being willing to 'place down' both ourselves and the outcomes of our actions, we succeed in reducing both egoism and attachment to the material aspects of life which are both obstacles to our progress in yoga. (p33 Religiousness in Yoga).

The third teaching on Īśvara Praṇidhānā is in chapter one verse twenty-three:

Īśvara-Praṇidhānā-va
Or surrender to Īśvara

Here the emphasis of the teaching rests on the qualities of Īśvara and the possibilities of surrendering to and linking with these qualities as a means of moving towards the state of yoga. The supreme qualities of Īśvara are detailed in sūtra 1:24-27. Īśvara is: '*viśeşah puruşa*' - a special/distinct puruşa/seer, superior to our own individual Seer. Īśvara is '*niratiśyaṃ*' - the highest, unsurpassed (intelligence). TKV Desikachar explains that these unique attributes allow Īśvara to perceive perfectly, unaffected by confusion and the ebb and flow of life (kleśa and karma). Īśvara is all knowing and able to see things we can't. Like the parent of a newly qualified young driver buying a cheap second-hand car who can see the forthcoming breakdowns and bills, whilst the young person can only see fun and freedom. Īśvara is also '*guruh kālena anavacchedāt*' – a timeless teacher, the first teacher, the teacher of all teachers and as such can be 'approached' to show the way. By linking with the qualities of Īśvara we come closer to understanding them and as our understanding grows we become more of these qualities ourselves.

Sutra 1:23 offers an alternative route to the rigours of the aṣṭāṅga yoga system given in chapter two. We are told, you can do all the work: physical practice, cultivate dispassion, adopt self-discipline, engage in ongoing self-study, practice yama, niyama, dhāraṇā etc., but there is another option: Īśvara Praṇidhānā – surrender to something higher. By simply surrendering to Īśvara, we can link to a greater wisdom than our own, perhaps of God, or the Universe, or Life, whatever you perceive 'something higher' to be. Through surrender it is possible to bypass our ego, our attachments, aversions, habit patterns and resistances and link with the flux and change of Life. This linking helps us feel confident and supported and move towards samādhi – the state of wholeness and integration.

The three sūtra on Īśvara Praṇidhānā offer us viewpoints which can help us towards a greater understanding of the whole. To re-cap, through contemplation of sūtra 2:1 we can consider Īśvara Praṇidhānā as acceptance, an acceptance that we cannot always control the outcomes of our actions and that therefore it is helpful to focus on the quality of our actions rather than the results. Using sūtra 2:45 we are able to explore Īśvara Praṇidhānā as acknowledgement of our place within the bigger picture and of Īśvara as something greater than ourselves. Then, working with sūtra 1:23 we can contemplate the superior qualities attributed to Īśvara, and Īśvara Praṇidhānā as a process of linking with these qualities in order to come closer to them ourselves.

Flowing harmoniously with Life using acceptance and awareness is a way of understanding Īśvara Praṇidhānā.

Orientation 5-10 mins

We begin this final study of the course by observing how the breath moves at the sternum/heart space. After practising, you may like to make notes on the qualities and directions of the breath-movements you observe.

Come into semi-supine position. Feel equal balanced on the floor. Allow the breath to flow through the nostrils.

Feel into the upper back and let the shoulder blades ease towards one another and down towards the back waist. Notice how this movement opens the chest.

Let the palms turn up to the ceilings, let the inner upper arms follow the same direction. Notice how this rotates the shoulders further back to the mat.

Now let your attention come onto the sternum and the attached ribs.

Observe any movements in the sternum and front ribs as you inhale.
4 breaths

What movements are there? In which directions?

What happens when you exhale? 4 breaths

Now let your attention come into the space behind the sternum. 4 breaths

What movement do you observe behind the sternum and ribs on each inhalation? On each exhalation? 4 breaths

Let your awareness come away from the sternum now. 2 breaths

How did you experience breath movements ***at*** *the sternum and ribs?*

How did it move? Directions?

Qualities?

Rough/smooth?

Long/short?

Consistent/changing?

Effortful/effortless?

How did you experience breath movements in the space ***behind*** *the sternum?*

How did it move? Directions?

Qualities?

Rough/ smooth?

Long/short?

Consistent/changing?

Effortful/effortless?

Īśvara Praṇidhānā: surrender

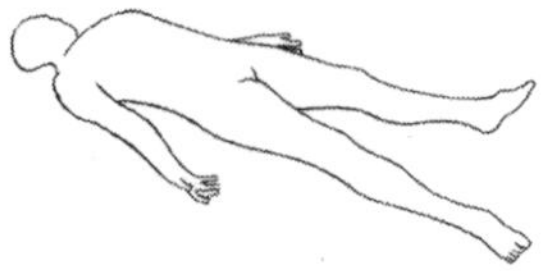

1. Savāsana – static

From semi-supine, stretch out arms then legs. Stay 6 breaths

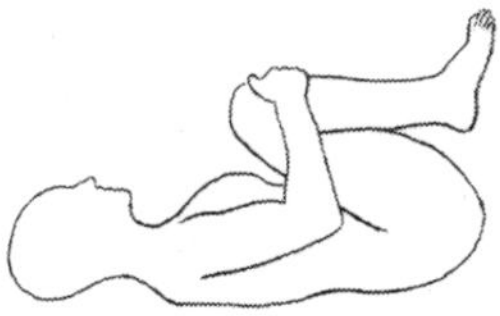

2. Apānāsana

Exhale draw knees into chest, inhale release x4

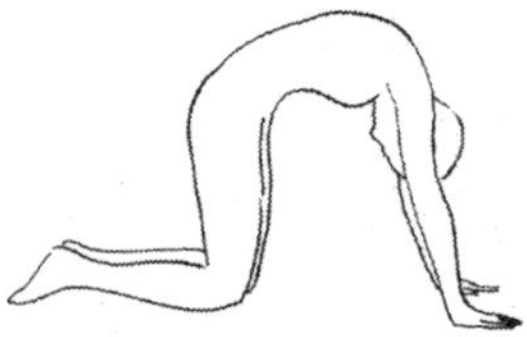

3. Cakravākāsana - dynamic

Inhale squeeze shoulder blades together, open chest

Exhale draw abdomen in and pull pelvis back from gripping fingertips

x4 rounds

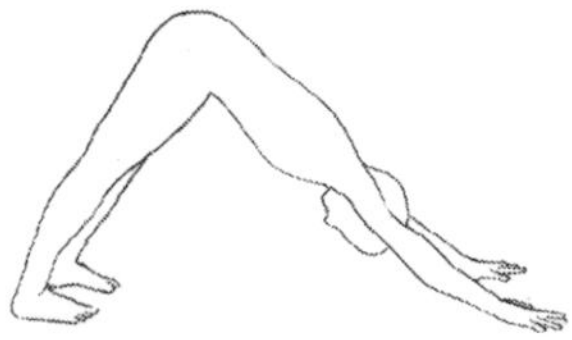

4. Adhomukha svānāsana - static

Inhale on all fours, exhale lift hips up and back

Stay - Inhale wide chest, exhale from lower abdomen

4-6 breaths, repeat

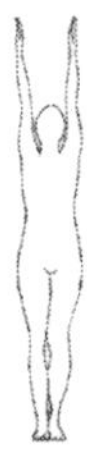

5. Tāḍāsana – static

Inhale raise arms, stay 4 breaths

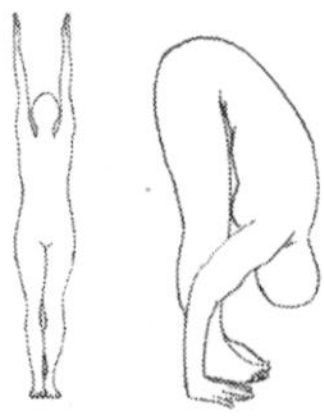

6. Ardha Uttānāsana/Uttānāsana - dynamic

Inhale raise arms, exhale fold forwards to 90' x4

Inhale raise arms, exhale full fold forwards x4

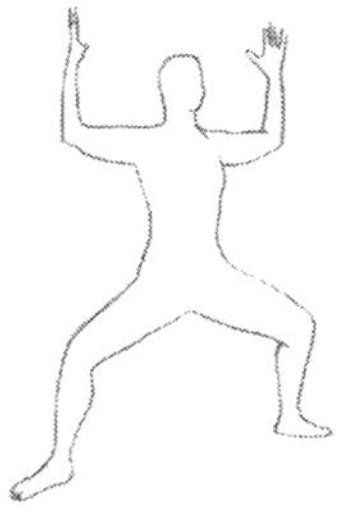

7. Prasārita Utkaṭāsana - static

Feet wide, inhale raise arms,
exhale bend knees and arms

Stay 4 breaths

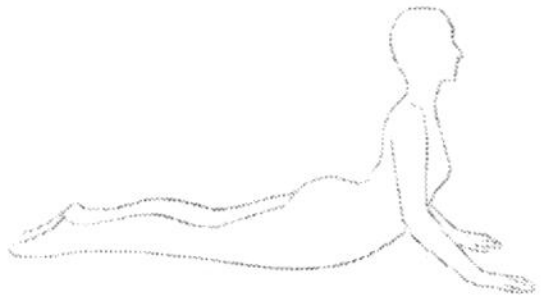

8. Bhujaṇgāsana - dynamic + static
Inhale raise chest, exhale lower x4
Lift and stay 4 breaths. Rest Balāsana

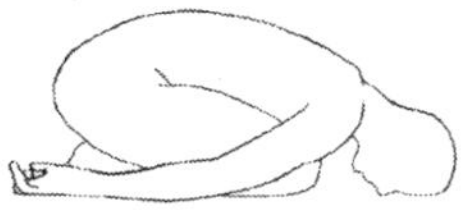

9. Balāsana – static
Stay 4 breaths

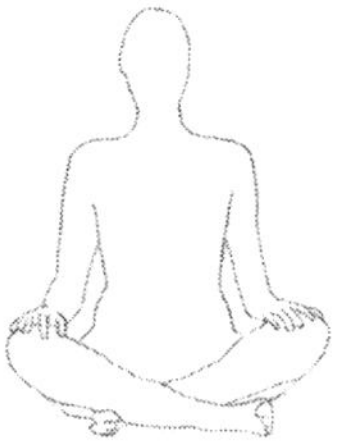

10. Sukhāsana – static

Stay 4-6 breaths

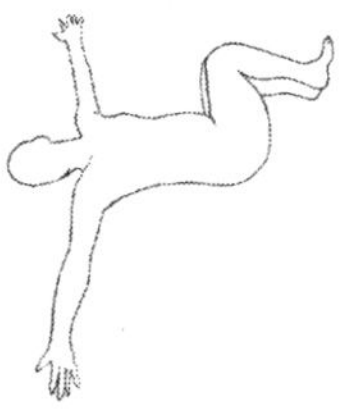

11. Jaṭhara parivṛtti – static

Exhale lower knees to floor
stay 4-6 breaths R + L

Counterpose – Apānāsana

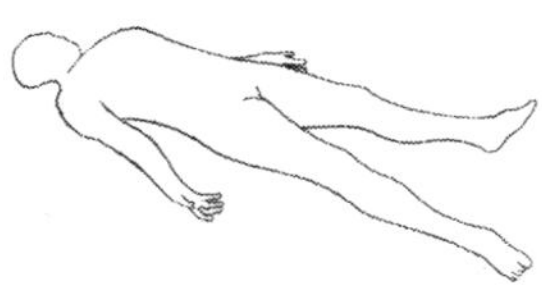

12. Savāsana - static

From semi-supine stretch out R leg then L

Stay 6 breaths.

1.Come into a comfortable seated position.

2. Revise breath counting technique.

3. Place R hand in Jñāna mudrā, left thumb ready at base of left forefinger to count.

4.Ujjāyī breathing with counting technique. 6 breaths

5. Teach Pratiloma Ujjāyī:

Inhale ujjāyī both nostrils. Exhale L single nostril. Inhale L single nostril. Exhale ujjāyī both nostrils

Inhale ujjāyī both nostrils. Exhale R single nostril. Inhale R single nostril. Exhale ujjāyī both nostrils

Continue with Pratiloma Ujjāyī using own breath length.
2 rounds/8 breaths

Check all ok.

6. Those who feel confident continue with Pratiloma Ujjāyī.
Others do Ujjāyī. 4 rounds/16 breaths

7. Release Ujjāyī. Simple breathing. 4 breaths

The focus for this practice is the qualities of Īśvara.

Come into a comfortable seated position, hands in Jñāna mudrā. 1 min

Lift and lengthen through the spine, create stability.

Let your awareness settle at the space behind the sternum, the place of Wisdom.

In the Indian system - the hṛdaya.

Bring to mind the qualities of Īśvara: unchanging, knower of all, seer of all, supreme teacher, special puruṣa.

Let your mind browse over them, then settle on one.

Hold it in your awareness. If the mind wanders gently bring it back. 5 mins

Let your attention gradually move back to your breathing.
1 min

Bring your hands together in the lap.
Gradually release your focus and lift your gaze.

Come out of the practice.

Īśvara Praṇidhānā - Surrender and Release

Lie in semi-supine or savāsana.

Feel that the body is in a comfortable position to release. Feel that the mind is in a mood to relax.

In this practice we will cultivate feelings of heaviness and softness in the body, encouraging it to feel heavy like sand or water or mud. We will give up any tension, any holding in the body and mind, allowing them to surrender and release into the ground.

Take your attention first into the feet. Begin to feel that the feet are becoming heavier and heavier. Heavy like sand, or water or mud. Each time you exhale, feel the heavy sand pour out through the soles of the feet. Feel it flow into the ground, releasing and relaxing as it goes, leaving the feet comfortable and soft and relaxed.

Now let your attention ease up into the legs, through the calves and shins, the knee joints and up into the thighs. Feel the legs becoming heavier and heavier like sand. Each time you exhale, the heavy sand releases from the backs of the legs and into the ground. As the heavy sand releases, the legs are becoming more and more released, leaving the legs comfortable soft and relaxed, surrendered into the support of the floor.

Now let your awareness travel into the pelvis. Become aware of the soft tissue of the abdominal muscles, the reproductive organs and the lower digestive tract. Become aware of the bony pelvic girdle. Feel the soft tissue and bony tissue becoming heavier and heavier. Imagine that the whole of the pelvis is filled with heavy sand. Now begin to feel that the sand is draining out through the centre of the back of the pelvis at the sacrum. The draining sand carries away any tension, any pain, any strain, leaving the whole pelvic area comfortable, soft and released into the ground.

Let your awareness travel up through the spine and into the thoracic cavity. Feel it becoming heavier and heavier. Imagine that the back of the thoracic cavity is heavy with sand. Each time you exhale the sand drifts away through the space between the shoulder blades. The upper spine, ribcage, heart and lungs are releasing with each out breath. The whole thoracic cavity is soft, comfortable and surrendered into the earth.

Allow your attention to travel along the collarbones and into the shoulders, arms, and hands. Feel them becoming heavier and heavier. Begin to imagine fine, heavy sand flowing out from the backs of the shoulders, the arms and the hands, carrying away any fatigue, strain or pain. Sand is steadily flowing out through the backs of the arms and hands leaving them soft, comfortable and releasing into the earth.

Now let your attention travel up into the head, to the back of the head where it rests perfectly poised on the floor. Begin to imagine that the head is becoming heavier and heavier, relaxing back into two hands which are gently supporting it. Let the muscles in the neck release, let the muscles in the face and jaw release, let the eye sockets soften. Feel that the head is becoming heavier and heavier and resting further and further back into the supporting hands. Surrender any holding in the head and neck. The face is soft and open and the eyes release back, dark and quiet. The whole head is released, the whole body is released. The whole body is released.

When the mind of a yogi is in harmony and rests in the Spirit within, all restless desires gone… His mind is a lamp whose light is steady, for it burns in a shelter where no winds come. Bhagavad Gītā 6:12

Rest quietly here for a few moments.

Let the feelings of relaxation and ease stay with you as you begin to become more aware of yourself resting.

Make small movements with fingers and toes.

Let your movements begin to grow and gradually reawaken your body in ways that you enjoy.

When you feel ready, rest onto your side for a few breaths before coming up to sitting.

Off the Mat Practices

Simplify everything you can.

Let go of as much 'stuff' as possible. Perhaps sort through your possessions asking 'Do I need this? Why?'

Act without any expectations of outcomes or reciprocity.

Read The Surrender Experiment, by Michael A. Singer

Plan from the basis of your present reality, not from a place of 'if…'

Go with the flow.

Become a gardener. Plant seeds, watch them grow.

Rent an allotment.

Sit quietly at a window once a day. Watch how the landscape changes.

Go for regular walks and observe changes in the environment.

Climb a high hill, clifftop or mountain. Wonder at the scope and perspective.

Gradually adjust your lifestyle to support your highest aspirations and health.

Live with purpose, awareness and understanding.

Cultivate an increased trust in the course of life.

Create the conditions to support your daily practice of yoga.
Release the things which get in the way of practice.

Contemplations

I release all attachments and desires.

Deep wisdom guides me.

The Wisdom of the Universe supports me.

I am awake to truth, peace and joy.

Things will never always be as I'd like them to be.

I surrender all expectations and trust.

How do you currently understand Īśvara Praṇidhānā?

Look back over your musings and notes for this course.

What do you feel you have made progress with?

What has become established?

What did you find difficult to grasp?

What did you try to do but found difficult to implement?

Part 5 - Conclusion

Ancient Teachings for the Modern Age

The Yoga Sūtra are steeped in ancient Indian traditions. Some aspects of ascetic practices, engaged in at that time, are evident within Patañjali's aṣṭāṅga system. For example, the fourth yama - brahmacharya (continence) and the third niyama - tapas (self-purification). However, within the eight-fold yoga system, austerities are practised thoughtfully, in moderation and not for their own sake. They are undertaken for the purpose of purifying the body and mind so that we might come closer towards mental clarity.

Niyama remain relevant and applicable for yoga practitioners, this is illustrated in the diagram below. Rather than a set of austere rules, niyama might be regarded as an intertwining mesh of supportive techniques. With sustained practice, they gradually spiral, refining the mind in the process. So for example, in the quietness of an āsana practice, we find that śauca (cleansing) takes place. Perhaps the small-stuff which had pre-occupied us settles and our priorities become clear. With greater awareness of what is important, we can cultivate an appreciation of what we already have (saṃtoṣa). At the simplest level, we value the degree of movement we enjoy, for the time and space to practice, for the training and knowledge given to us. Śauca and saṃtoṣa within the process of practice bring qualities of openness, spaciousness and balance - sattva guṇa is present.

The clarity of sattva helps us recognise changes which need to be made: old habits which should be let go; the value of a better diet, consistent sleep patterns and regular exercise (tapas). Through tapas we make these changes and gain stability. In turn stability assists self-study (svādhyāya) then greater self-understanding re-supports tapas by illuminating further aspects which require improvement, for example our speech/communication. Such growing awareness supports us towards Īśvara Praṇidhānā – recognising our place within the 'bigger picture'. In turn, Īśvara Praṇidhānā nourishes contentment and mental purity. More sattva arises, its clarity carries us steadily on and the spiralling interplay of niyama continues. Together with the remaining seven limbs, and supported by practice and dispassion, niyama guide us ever closer towards the harmony of samādhi.

I wish you well in your practice.

		Integration/Samadhi	
		↑	
		clarity	
		sattva	
		↑	
A	**self-purification**	**self-study**	**surrender**
B	tapas	svādhyāya	Īśvara Praṇidhānā
H		**clarity**	
Y		sattva	
Ā		↑	
S	**self-purification**	**self-study**	**surrender**
A	tapas	svādhyāya	Īśvara Praṇidhānā
+		↑	
V		**clarity**	
A		sattva	
I		↑	
R			
Ā		**cleanliness + contentment**	
G		śauca + saṃtoṣa	
Y		↑	
A		**cleanliness**	
		śauca	

Abhyāsa: practice. Vairāgya: dispassion

Final Reflections

You may find it useful to consider ways of applying the teachings on niyama which you have studied. How might you develop each element in your life? Perhaps note down one practical way for each:

Śauca external:

Śauca internal:

Saṃtoṣa:

Tapas:

Svādhyāya:

Īśvara Praṇidhānā:

Part 6 - Resources

Bibliography

Bouanchaud B. 1997 The Essence of Yoga Sri Satguru Publications. Delhi.

Chapple C and Kelly E.P. 1990 The Yoga Sutras of Patañjali Sri Satguru Publications. Delhi.

Charlton David and Roy Ranju 2019 Embodying The Yoga Sūtra, YogaWords, Pinter and Martin, London

Desikachar TKV 1995 The Heart Of Yoga Inner Traditions International. Vermont.

Desikachar TKV 1980 Religiousness in Yoga University Press of America. London.

Desikachar TKV 2001 In Search of Mind. Second Edition Krishnamacharya Yoga Mandarin. Chennai.

Easwaren Eknath 1985 The Bhagavad Gītā Nilgiri Press. California.

Farhi D 2000 Yoga Mind, Body and Spirit Newleaf. Dublin.

Feuerstein Georg 1990 Encyclopedic Dictionary of Yoga , Paragon House USA.

Feuerstein Georg 2003 The Deeper Dimension of Yoga Shambala. Boston.

Harvey P 2001 Yoga For Everybody Time-Life Books. London

Isherwood C and Prabhavananda Swami 1953 How To Know God Vedanta Press. California.

Krafstow G 1999 Yoga For Wellness Compass Penguin. New York.

Levine Stephen 1979 A Gradual Awakening. Anchor Books. USA

Lloyd Gill 2015 Yoga: The Early Story Lulu Enterprises. New York

Mascaro Juan 1962 The Bhagavad Gītā Penguin. London.

Mohan A G 1993 Yoga For Body breath and Mind Shambala. London.

Mohan A G and Indra 2004 Yoga Therapy Shambala (London)

Nataraja Shanida 2008 The Blissful Brain: Neuroscience and proof of the power of meditation. Gaia. London

Ramaswami Srivatsa and Hurwitz D 2006 Yoga Beneath The Surface Marlowe and Company, New York.

Satchidananda Swami 1978 The Yoga Sutras of Patañjali Intergral Yoga Publications. Virginia.

Sargeant Winthrop 2009 The Bhagavad Gita State University New York Press, Albany.

Shearer Alistair 1982 The Yoga Sutras of Patañjali Random House. New York.

Sturgess Stephen 2002 The Yoga Book Watkins Publishing. London.

About The Author

Susan Lodge MA (Ed), PGCE, BA, BWY Diploma, YFHF Cert.

Ongoing postgraduate study with Paul Harvey:

1:1: on going personal practice development, Yoga Sūtra study.

Modules: Asana, Hatha Yoga Energetics, Sound and Chanting, Bhagavad Gītā, Upanishads, Yoga Sūtra of Patañjali, Ayurveda, Samkhya.

Susan offers:

- 1-1 personal lessons for practice and health support
- Small group courses for personal development and preparation for professional training
- BWY CPD on the teachings of Patanjali's Yoga Sutra
- Yoga Planning Handbooks for students and teachers
- Relaxation weekends - www.greataytonlodge.co.uk

I welcome enquiries or general contact to discuss any aspects of the above:
yogasusanlodge@outlook.com

Forthcoming Titles in the 'Handbooks for Yoga Practice' Series:

Kriyā Yoga

Śraddhā

Kleśa

Obstacles to Progress

Abhyāsa and Vairāgya